Information about the myriad causes of vulvovaginal pain is hard to find in the world of caring clinicians. Education about normal female sexual function is not robust. Imagine the challenges of a woman looking for help for both vulvovaginal pain *and* pain with sex. And what about the challenges of the clinician trying to help—what do you prescribe?

Clinicians do not usually prescribe pleasure to treat pain.

Welcome the long-needed combination of a savvy and talented sex educator and coach, Elizabeth Wood, with Dee Hartmann, a wise and gifted physical therapist specializing in pelvic floor muscle problems. In *The Pleasure Prescription*, they have teamed up to help with both sources of suffering in women.

The book compares pleasure and pain as two sides of a coin, but this coin does not get flipped. Physical therapy muscle work is blended with equal parts of pleasuring from somatic sex education. For a woman who understands both sides of the coin, who continues treatment for any persistent vulvovaginal problem, help is on the way.

—Elizabeth G. Stewart, MD, FACOG
Director Emerita, The V Service Atrius Health,
Boston, Massachusetts
Author, *The V Book*, and co-author,
vulvovaginal disorders.org

The lived experience of authors Hartmann and Wood, as colleagues who successfully treat women with chronic vulvovaginal pain or pain with sex, has led them to a radical concept: that the ongoing and burgeoning experience of pleasure can alter and heal pain. This is not a concept that fits into the "medical model" of fixing what is broken about the body. The concept reassures women who experience sexual pain that, whatever their medical diagnosis, *dysfunction* is not a word that will be used to describe them. Through deeper understanding of their own bodies, especially the trusting and flowering experience of pleasure, women with pain will be able to gradually heal themselves.

As clinicians who treat women with vulvovaginal complaints, including sexual pain or the inability to have sex, we are aware of the complexity of the structures that meet at the female vulva. We also understand the complexity of human thoughts and emotions tied to these areas of the body. We see the suffering women and their families are experiencing, but we do not have the tools to help if salves and pills don't work. Those of us who have become vulvovaginal specialists know that many of our patients finally improve when we send them to an experienced pelvic floor physical therapist, but we don't know how that happens. The combined knowledge in this book of a sexuality educator and pelvic floor physical therapist begins to let us in on the secrets they have discovered over their many years of practice.

—Ione Bissonnette,
nurse midwife and vulvovaginal specialist
Co-author of www.vulvovaginaldisorders.org

This is an excellent read for any woman who has ever struggled with sexual pain. Not only is there a wealth of information, but *The Pleasure Prescription* is an easy and enjoyable read. The writing style is witty and extremely relatable for anyone who has ever struggled with this kind of pain. Each chapter explores a real struggle experienced by a patient of one of the authors and includes a recommendation at the end, with excellent suggestions for combatting your pain using pleasant or pleasurable touch. Most of the recommendations delve into getting to know your own vulva and vagina through touch and what feels good to you. As you learn and grow through the information in each chapter, the recommendations build and change with you. The authors discuss many important topics that all women experience when it comes to their sexual health. And the reader feels validated and understood in their struggle with sexual pain. This book is definitely a must-read.

—National Vulvodynia Association

The *Pleasure* Prescription

A Surprising Approach to
Healing Sexual Pain

Dee Hartmann, PT, DPT, IF and
Elizabeth Wood, MSW, CSSE, CTE, BC

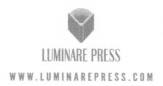

LUMINARE PRESS
WWW.LUMINAREPRESS.COM

*Dee Hartmann: To my best friend and husband,
David, for loving and supporting me enough to say, "I can't
believe you did all that weird stuff in your practice all those
years only to start doing something even weirder."*

*Elizabeth Wood: To my father, Peter H. Wood,
who made it possible for me to follow my own path.
As a "proper" English gentleman, you were never comfortable
"discussing such matters," yet you were always there
to support and encourage my journey.*

Contents

PART ONE

The Introductory Practices

PART TWO

The Advanced Solo Practices

PART THREE

The Partnered Practices

A Note from Our Lawyers

Hey, this should be obvious, but just in case:

We are professional educators who provide information in the area of human sexuality. Though you may find some of the information in this book to be therapeutic, we are not licensed psychotherapists or medical doctors, and we are not providing psychotherapy services or medical help through this book.

More specifically, our lawyers insist that we tell you that any information found within these pages is not intended to treat, diagnose, test, assign, or counsel any individual or group for the purpose of alleviating mental disorders; understanding unconscious or conscious motivation; resolving emotional, relationship, or attitudinal conflicts; or modifying behaviors that interfere with effective emotional, social, or intellectual functioning. They also want you to know that the information you read here is also not intended to diagnose, treat, or cure any disease (but we're pretty sure you knew that…right?). And we agree wholeheartedly that if you need psychotherapy services or medical help you should absolutely seek out the assistance of a licensed professional right away.

We do both have extensive career histories working with women, and you'll find some of these women's stories in the chapters to follow. Since we were acting in a professional capacity, we are required (both legally and ethically) to protect our patients' and clients' confidentiality. Because of this, all names and identifying details have been changed, and on several occasions, we've combined key details from similar stories in order to represent the most typical cases we've seen. So if we've worked with you one-on-one, don't worry; your vulva, and your secrets, are safe with us.

Preface

A Note from Elizabeth:

Over the last number of years, I have been both a student and teacher of a most profound subject: women's sexual pleasure. Having discovered my own personal pleasures, I began to share the wealth of this accumulated knowledge of pleasure with my clients. The results were extraordinary—and particularly so with a specific set of clients. Over time, the clients who had come to me describing pain with sex began to report that their pain was decreasing. Not only that, but they were feeling happier too. Was I on to something? Could pleasure be part of the conundrum of sexual pain?

The answers were yes, but it felt like I only had half the equation. While I had long considered myself a pleasure crusader—almost a renegade, alone in a field without others who saw the world through this pleasure lens—I wasn't an expert in helping women alleviate unwanted sexual pain. I was like Laverne without Shirley, Thelma without Louise— or, for the even younger of you, our dear readers, Lorelai without Rory.

There was just one person I could call to accompany me on the journey that lay ahead. I needed someone, herself a renegade in her field, to form an extraordinary dynamic duo like no other.

A Note from Dee:

It was a quintessential summer morning. I sat in my rocking chair, enjoying the view across the lake. After nearly thirty years, I had just retired from clinical practice. I was no longer Dee Hartmann, Physical Therapist, who thought about things like which pelvic floor exercises to prescribe; I was now Dee Hartmann, Full-Time Grandma, and I was thinking about all the free time I would be spending with my five grandbabies. I sipped my morning coffee and envisioned what was to come: hearing the grandbabies coo, changing dirty diapers, cleaning up goo, and juggling nap schedules (the grandbabies', not mine!). I let myself get lost in the happy future that awaited me. I looked out over the lake. I had waited a long time for this.

Then the phone rang.

It was Elizabeth, my former colleague and longtime friend. If I expected to hear congratulations on a well-earned retirement, I was quickly disappointed. "You can't retire, Dee!" she insisted. "At least not yet. There's more we have to do, and we're the only ones who can do it. We have to take our message out into the world, and we have to do it together!" Over the course of my career, I had become an expert in treating women's sexual pain. And I knew what she was saying was true. With over fifty years of combined experience on opposite ends of women's sexual health and wellness, we had often discussed a revolutionary conclusion: our two areas of expertise, sexual pain and sexual pleasure, were two sides of the same coin. Treating one would affect the other. While it was obvious that the less pain a woman feels, the more pleasure she can experience, no one seemed to be talking about what Elizabeth had first identified to me, which I had then confirmed over and over in my practice: that increasing pleasure has the potential to decrease pain.

I sighed as I looked deeper into the lake. Elizabeth was right. We needed to start a new, fresh conversation on women's sexual health and wellness—one that no one else seemed to be having. The only question was: how was I going to cofound a women's pleasure movement, write a book, and still have time for all those grandbabies? But I was in.

That phone call marked the first step toward our Pleasure Movement and the birth of our first company, VulvaLove, Inc. (www.vulvalove.com), which educates women about their bodies and sexual pleasure. Our next goal was to write *The Pleasure Prescription*. From there, it was a natural progression to formally launch the Pleasure Movement™ (www.pleasuremovement.com).

Since *The Pleasure Prescription* has two authors, we debated on how to refer to ourselves. From this point forward, we'll write in what is technically called the first-person plural, meaning we refer to ourselves as "we," and we'll refer to ourselves in the third-person singular ("Elizabeth" and "Dee") whenever we need to be more specific. While we agree on pretty much everything you'll read here, you'll find "Notes from Elizabeth" and "Notes from Dee" throughout the book. These reflect our individual thoughts and suggestions, which most often come from our professional points of view.

With that, let us formally introduce ourselves, along with a little background on how we came to those professional opinions.

Elizabeth is an expert in pleasure. After receiving a master's degree in social work in 1998, she was a licensed therapist for many years, specializing in sex therapy. But the longer she worked as a sex therapist, the more frustrated she became by the medicalization of female sexual dysfunction. As she saw it, the medical model paid no attention to women's lack of experience, connection to their bodies, or to their sexuality. So, in 2012, Elizabeth willingly gave up her license and walked away from the traditional world of sex therapy. It was then that she began to study comprehensive, evidence-based, sex-positive sex education; somatic healing; tantra; spiritual sexuality; and other modalities addressing sexual healing. Her learning took her far outside of academic textbooks and further into a more holistic way of helping women with the problems they had with their bodies and sexuality. She explored pleasure and the female orgasm extensively. Today, she provides sexual education and healing resources through workshops, public speaking, and private coaching sessions to women and couples from a wide range of backgrounds.

Dee has been a practicing physical therapist for over forty years. After enrolling her fifth child in kindergarten, she opened her private practice. For the more than two decades that followed, she worked with women to help them understand, address, and alleviate issues with chronic pelvic and abdominal pain, problems with bowel and bladder control, and chronic problems with vulvar pain that typically lead to painful or impossible sex. Since opening one of the first women's health physical therapy private practices in the Chicagoland area, Dee has worked tirelessly to educate physicians and other medical professionals. Her goal has been to raise awareness of pelvic floor physical therapy as an adjunct to traditional patient care. (Even so, there are still gynecologists and general practitioners who aren't familiar with the specialty, so don't feel bad if you've never heard of it either!) In addition to her clinical work, she has published and lectured to professionals around the world as an expert in women's sexual health. Despite her retirement from clinical practice, Dee continues to speak at medical meetings. Her talks include the importance of *increased pleasure* as an integral part of a healthy, pain-free lifestyle.

The two of us met in 2004 when we were chosen as team members to open a new women's sexual dysfunction center. We hit it off right away and knew that in each other we'd met our sexual health kindred spirit. Though we only worked together a short time at the new clinic, our friendship continued to grow as we went off in our own professional directions. Throughout the years, we relied on each other, often consulting together on our most difficult cases. Our calls were enriching, providing us deeper insight to better serve the women in our respective private practices.

We began to discuss our discomfort with the medicalization of women's sexual health. Although the medical model classifies a number of women's sexual health issues and problems as dysfunctions, we never chose to identify our clients as dysfunctional. For us, a medical approach to women's sexual health had not adequately addressed the needs and concerns of our clients—including many women who have pain with sex. In our own practices, we each took a different approach. We saw women as whole beings who weren't broken and didn't need to be fixed, so our methodology was to teach women how to heal themselves. We started teaching them how their bodies worked and then guided them to feel deep inside. From there, most were able to solve their own problems—which we believe is far more effective than us attempting to solve them.

This approach isn't common. In fact, the sexual health community has medicalized women's sexual health to the point of dysfunction. While there are studies, diagnoses, and treatments regarding women's sexual dysfunction, relatively few address women's sexual function and education, and there is very little focus on pleasure. Most women, and many of the doctors who treat them, lack extensive education around female arousal, orgasm, and women's sexuality as a whole—let alone how pleasure can help decrease pain. Though we've surely been looking, we've never met a medical doctor who prescribes pleasure and/or arousal to help improve or reverse symptoms of pain; in fact, though the female reproductive system is as geared toward pleasure as it is toward reproduction, pleasure isn't typically a part of the medical conversation in reference to women's sexual health.

And the pain we're referencing here goes beyond just physical pain. Women commonly feel pain with sex, pain with arousal, and pain at their vulvas when doing simple things such as inserting a tampon or wearing underwear. This is often accompanied by the psychological pain that comes with feeling they're alone in their physical pain—an unfortunate reality, because as we both know, pain is common. The pain multiplies from there. Some women feel ashamed that they're not that interested in sex; others are devastated that they've never had an orgasm or mortified that it takes them so long to reach one. Women feel the pain of hating their bodies, of not knowing what turns them on, and, quite often, the pain of *feeling like they're missing out on something.* That thing is pleasure, and its lack brings immeasurable emotional pain—which, in turn compounds any physical symptoms they have.

We wrote this book to address women's sexual pain, both physical and emotional, from a broader standpoint: one that puts pleasure front and center. And we truly believe that what we have to offer is nothing short of revolutionary.

Introduction

Something strange is going on with women's sexual pain. Though the issue is common and well-documented, many women spend years searching for a diagnosis and even longer searching for a solution. Sexual pain can be hard to talk about, confusing to address, and utterly demoralizing for those who face it. And frankly, the way many of us are treating this problem—including the women who suffer from it, the medical community that addresses it (or doesn't), and society at large—just isn't working.

So why isn't it working? Well, we can start by looking at the angle from which women's sexual pain is most often approached. Those who practice using the traditional medical model generally know how something works before they try to fix it. However, when it comes to female sexual function, most of the available research and financial resources are directed in the opposite way—toward how to fix sexual dysfunction rather than understand normal functioning. From a research perspective, we don't fully know what normal sexual function is! A debate still rages over the nature and origin of the female orgasm as well as the function and anatomy of the entire female sexual arousal network. And what we do know about pleasure isn't focused on women. Historically, research has been directed predominantly toward the study of men's bodies and male sexual dysfunction, with the findings then applied to female sexual dysfunction.

As we stated in the Preface, our conversations began when we realized we were approaching women's sexual health from two separate angles. But though our professional backgrounds are so different, we found that many of our clients had been diagnosed by their medical practitioners with female sexual dysfunction. As we saw it, many of them weren't actually dysfunctional; they certainly were dealing with issues, challenges, and problems, but there wasn't anything physically wrong with them. What they were lacking—sexual pleasure and sufficient arousal states—was never part of the conversation with their medical providers. Many of our clients simply had no interest in sex, but when we questioned them further, many of them didn't understand how arousal, pleasure, or even their very own bodies worked. We're pretty well-educated and quite accustomed to talking about sex, so from our vantage point, this was yet another tragedy. In fact, we were downright incensed by this reality. It seemed utterly unfair that women possessed such high capacity for pleasure and yet were so often unable to access it.

This was part of a greater issue across the country, and likely the world: the *orgasm gap*. As it turns out, women have fewer orgasms than men—a lot fewer. Evidence shows that heterosexual women, in particular, have as few as one orgasm for every three their male partners experience. They also experience less pleasure in general. And this is despite the fact that it's much easier for females to have multiple orgasms than it is for males. There are a whole lot of reasons for this. For one, many people think of sex as something that ends when a man comes. Mainstream pornography hammers this idea in: it's rarely focused on women's pleasure; it usually ends with a man ejaculating; and the number of female orgasms versus male orgasms filmed is, quite frankly, abysmal. Unfortunately, a lot of people's sex lives mirror this, meaning a lot of women don't come even though their partners do. Most of us, men and women included, haven't been taught that there's anything wrong with this. The orgasm gap isn't just a statistical issue—it's an issue that we have seen over and over in our professional lives. And we refuse to believe it is simply the byproduct of female dysfunction.

So we decided on a plan. First, we created a method to work through pain that increased women's *sexual agency*: their sense of authority or ownership over their own bodies and their own pleasure. And then we began to take women through the steps of creating or restoring a healthy, amazing, enjoyable relationship with sex. All along the way, we advocated practices and attitudes that are *pleasure-forward*—our term for prioritizing pleasure and letting it dominate the experience. And it worked. We found that most of our clients were able to make gains toward better sexual health.

As we see it, our prescription starts with education, moves through guided self-exploration, and eventually graduates to partnered experience. This is how we can guide pleasure to overtake pain.

And that, dear reader, is precisely what this book aims to do.

About This Book

This book starts with "Part I: The Introductory Practices," which aims to teach you about how your body works and explore its capacity to feel, including both pain and pleasure. The exercises, which we call *prescriptions*, are simple in this section, yet we've seen throughout our careers that these experiences alone have the power to change women's lives. "Part II: The Advanced Solo Practices" builds upon the themes explored in Part I by taking a deeper dive into what makes you unique and amazing as pleasure begins to run the show. This requires moving from exploration into practice, preparing for "Part III: The Partnered Practices," which allows you to bring what you've learned to a partner, if you so choose.

And this piece is important, because not everyone wants to share this with a partner—and many don't have a partner to share it with! We absolutely understand that. If you are partnered, we encourage you to read through the third section and consider whether it's right for you to bring what you learn into your shared bed. If you are unpartnered by choice, you may choose to skip the third section, or just skim through it to get any juicy bits and add them to your pleasure repertoire. And if you aren't partnered, but want to be, consider the third section a roadmap for the relationship you hope to create in the future.

Throughout all three sections, we hope to inspire you to better understand the value of your own pleasure. One of our main goals is to help you see *that you are worthy of pleasure*. You deserve to feel good. You deserve the sex life of your dreams. You deserve to enjoy life, both in and out of the bedroom, on your own and/or with a partner. To help you get there, we are providing the sex education that you didn't get in grammar school—education that is focused on pleasure, or as we like to say, *pleasure-forward*, rather than focused on reproduction, anatomy, and disease.

Each chapter begins with a story from one of Dee's patients or Elizabeth's clients. Then we spend the bulk of the chapter looking at the main things we discussed with her and end the chapter with a few prescriptions for home practice. The ten women represented in this book have problems that are common; each of them was dealing with issues that we've seen many women face over the course of our careers. But we want to be clear: each woman is complex, and it is rare that a single prescription will help her feel better overall. Some of these women saw us for a while, and some saw us for less time, but nearly all received quite a few prescriptions in the process—just as you are receiving a multilevel *Pleasure Prescription* in this book. In all cases, it was not our goal to "fix" the women who came to us for help; rather, we guided them through the process of addressing their own sexual well-being.

That brings us to the level of sexual well-being we're discussing within these pages. We assume you understand the meaning of the phrase "the birds and the bees," and we're not educating you on how all that works. Instead, we want you to understand that women are uniquely equipped for pleasure. As a matter of fact, women are hardwired for pleasure and have a specific body part—the clitoris—whose sole function is to provide sexual pleasure. This book will help you take advantage of that fact and use it to improve…well, pretty much everything about your life.

We'll provide tools to help you have better sex and increase your overall sense of self, which we believe go hand-in-hand. It's

congratulations! Way to go! We're so proud of you, and we just know you can do it.

The truth is we want this book to fuel our movement, the Pleasure Movement. Because here's what lies at the heart of what we believe: *happy, well-pleasured, empowered women will be in less pain…and eventually, they'll be able to make the world a better place.* It's a tall order, but one we are confident we can help create with this book. Read on. We have so much more in store for you.

Part One

The Introductory Practices

CHAPTER ONE

Getting to Know Your Body

A Note from Elizabeth:

> *Jaime was a typical client in her mid-thirties. She came to me with the same complaints I'd heard dozens of times before: she didn't like sex—or, well, she did, but not as much as she thought she should, and certainly not as much as her partner liked it. During our introductory call, she told me her partner was always the one to initiate sex, not because she was ashamed to do so but because she just rarely thought about it. She admitted that she might have climaxed once or twice back in college but barely remembered what it was like, let alone how to make it happen again. As Jaime described it, she just wasn't that into sex. "Am I missing out on something?" she asked.*
>
> *I encouraged Jaime to book a session for the following week.*
>
> *Before she came into my office, I emailed Jaime an assessment form. I send these to all new clients, who typically respond with surprise that I ask such personal questions before meeting face to face. But my clients quickly find out that if they're going to work with me, they're going to have to get down to the nitty-gritty right away. The assessment asks about arousal levels, the types of stimulation they enjoy, if they climax, and if so, both how and how often, etc. In Jaime's case, she reported low levels of arousal, that she rarely thought about sex, was distraught she couldn't climax, and disliked oral sex. She just wanted to have an orgasm with "normal"*

sex. If she could fix her body to do that, she wrote on the form, she might like sex a little bit more.

It was clear that Jaime wasn't aroused or experiencing climax with the sex she was having. But instead of changing what was going on during sex, she was hoping she could just change herself. She thought there was something wrong with her. From what I could tell, she knew very little about what felt good to her and held little value for her own pleasure. What she wanted was to have an orgasm during penetration. She thought this would make her feel normal.

One of the last questions on my assessment form is: How do you feel about the way your vulva looks? On a scale of 0–10, Jaime answered "3," which was below a neutral "5." From that answer alone, I knew genital education was the place to start.

There's a lot going on for Jaime, and all of it is fairly common—actually, really common. In our experience, we have encountered countless women with one major complaint: they don't enjoy sex. Most of these define *sex* as having a penis in their vagina and call it "normal sex." Everything else is either "foreplay" or "something I do on my own" (Dee notes that it is extremely rare, in her line of work, to hear anyone—patient or practitioner—use the words *masturbate* or *self-pleasure*). In fact, studies have shown that many women are deeply focused on the male orgasm; over half of them consider it very important that their partner ejaculates during intercourse.[1] While speaking at a college campus, we asked the women in the audience how they defined "satisfactory sex," and several responded "when my partner comes."

Why didn't they think of their own pleasure? Upon further questioning, many admitted they had no understanding of how their bodies worked. They know they've got *stuff*, they just don't know *what that stuff does*—or how to make it work. And to take it a step further, many were hiding a dark and shameful secret: they

Dee Hartmann and Elizabeth Wood

truly didn't like their vulvas. As one woman noted, "It looks weird, smells funny, and it doesn't do what it's supposed to do."

When we encounter a woman in this situation, the first thing we have to do is teach her about her own anatomy. That's the purpose of this chapter: to teach you about typical female anatomy, focusing on what Sheri Winston, author of *Women's Anatomy of Arousal*, calls the *arousal network*.[2] The female arousal network is a web of tissues, organs, and glands that provide a series of functions (including things like blood engorgement and muscular tension and release), all of which are working toward a singular purpose: your pleasure. What does this mean? It means that this entire network is there to make you feel good—like really, really good.

Depending on how you were parented and what kind of sexual education you received, if any, you may know quite a bit about your reproductive system: the fallopian tubes, the uterus, the menstrual cycle, etc. But the female arousal network? Knowledge about *that* is far less common. So chances are, most of this stuff will be new to you—and that's totally okay. You're here to learn.

The truth is that most sex ed falls short of being…well, *sexual*. It's more like disease prevention and reproductive education. And that's only if the school provides sex ed; as of this writing, only twenty-four states and the District of Columbia require public schools to teach sex ed, and only ten of those mandate that it should be medically, factually, or technically accurate![3] Even when it *is* medically accurate, you can bet it's not pleasure-forward. Most sex ed teaches young people how to avoid pregnancy and disease. Very few people are explicitly taught about arousal and pleasure.

Over the years, we've found that very few people have any knowledge of *what* the female arousal network *is*, let alone know *how it works*. Most women grow up learning that we shouldn't look at or touch ourselves—let alone enjoy anything our vulvas and vaginas have to offer. We know that education is key for women to feel comfortable exploring their sexual capacity. As Elizabeth says, "You don't buy a Porsche without an owner's manual, yet I don't know anyone who has an owner's manual for their own body."

This chapter provides one. It's an owner's manual for your body. Here, we'll offer you a primer on your anatomy, and specifically the anatomy relating to your arousal network, on both the outside (your vulva) and the inside (your vagina). We'll describe what's normal and what isn't. (Spoiler alert: We'll assure you that most of it *is normal.*) At the end of the chapter, we'll ask you to take a look at yourself to see what's going on, you know, *down there.* We'll send you for a trip, with a mirror, to look at your own vulva. But first, we'll explain what you are likely to see when you get there.

External Anatomy

Let's start with the exterior parts of your arousal network: your vulva. The *vulva* refers to an area of tissues that extends from the pubic bone on the top to the sitz bones (ischial tuberosity) below.

Most of us have seen a diagram of the vulva. If you were in a basic sex ed class in school, you've likely seen the diagram of a vulva that we're about to show you. Sadly, for many women, the diagram is the only vulva they've ever seen. And there's another big problem with this particular diagram: it's just a graphic and lacks little resemblance to what's actually between a woman's legs. This has left many women who've only ever seen this diagram thinking something about their vulva is *wrong.* This is, of course, not the case, because just like faces, *vulvas are amazingly diverse.* (How diverse? Keep reading; we'll get there toward the end of the chapter.) In any case, we think that this "textbook vulva" diagram can do a lot of damage to women's self-esteem, so we use it purposefully.

With all that said, here's the diagram of the textbook vulva. We're using it to point out what and where everything is. Your vulva and all its parts will look different from what's in the picture. Each vulva will be different in color, size, and shape. The exact location and measurement of each part will differ too. Your parts may appear more or less symmetrical in one area or another. And that's all completely normal.

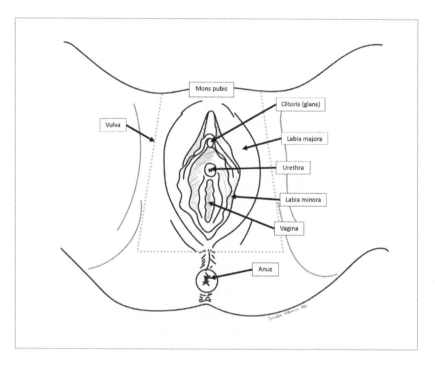

*That, friends, is one version of a vulva.
We call her the "textbook vulva."*

Let's take it from the top. Above the pubic bone is the area where pubic hair grows from puberty onward. This is called the *mons pubis.* It will vary in color and fullness from woman to woman, and it contains oil-secreting glands that release substances that are involved in sexual attraction, also known as *pheromones.*[4] Because it has anatomic connections to areas below that respond to sexual stimulation, stimulating the mons may also provide arousal. But for the purpose of this lesson, we're going to consider the mons pubis to be the very edge of the arousal network—like the suburbs, not the main city.

The pubic hair then extends down the sides of the vulva and sometimes down the thighs. You may or may not have pubic hair on your vulva, depending on your age and whether you prefer having it there or not. The rounded, squishy lips of flesh on the outer side are called the *outer labia*, or *labia majora*. They contain glands that produce sweat and oil, thus providing lubrication.[5] Inside the outer labia are the *inner labia*, or *labia minora*. This is the second set of lips, which are made of a much more sensitive type of skin, and which do not grow hair. Beneath that skin, there are all sorts of nerve endings that can make touch feel really good. There are also a whole lot of blood vessels, which, when you're aroused, become engorged, which means filled with blood. This engorgement causes them to swell up and become more sensitive to stimulation.[6]

When the labia are spread apart, you can see the *vaginal opening*. All things entering or leaving the vagina do so through the vaginal opening. It's a round orifice made of soft, moist mucus membrane that leads to the vaginal canal. We'll talk more about the vagina in a bit.

With the lips still spread, look above the entrance to the vagina and you'll see a small opening that leads to the *urethra*. It may be a bit difficult to see at first. The urethra is, in short, where your pee comes out. We don't consider the urethral opening to be a part of the arousal network, as touching or rubbing it doesn't give pleasure to most women we've encountered. In fact, any prolonged contact of the urethra can cause pain, irritation, and possibly urinary tract infections.

The labia minora come together to form a hood of tissue (more on this on the next page) that covers the shaft of the clitoris and the *clitoral glans*, often called the *clitoris* or *clit*. As we'll explain shortly, the clitoris is actually much larger than just the glans; the glans is the end of the clitoral shaft and the only external, visible part. And it's absolutely power-packed with nerve endings.[7] There are approximately seven to eight thousand sensory nerve endings in the clitoris. That's the exact same range that can be found in the penis; however, relative to the penis, clitoral nerve endings are packed into one-tenth the area. The clitoral glans contains several different types of nerve endings, including ones that code light touch (Merkel's discs), deep touch (Pacinian corpuscles), and skin stretch (Ruffini's nerve endings). This means the clitoris is incredibly sensitive to a wide variety of touch. And, when the clitoris becomes engorged with blood due to varying touch, magical things happen; you'll read plenty about that in the pages to come.

Now, back to the fold of skin covering the clitoris, which may or may not obscure the clitoris from view, depending on the woman's individual anatomy and level of arousal. This is called the *clitoral hood*. For most women, touching and rubbing the clitoral hood feels good, as it provides indirect stimulation of the glans beneath it. For many women, this is a fabulous option; sometimes direct clitoral stimulation can be too intense.

Once you've located the vaginal opening, look for the *anus* below, which is where bowel movements exit our bodies. Between the anus and the vaginal opening, you'll see a bridge of tissue that is called the *perineal body*. Some women feel sexual pleasure when this area is stimulated.

So, that's everything on the outside that you can see. Let's look at what's inside, because there's a whole lot more to your arousal network.

Internal Anatomy

We'll start with the vagina. As we covered in the Introduction, the vagina is actually a very precise part of the body—it's not the vulva itself. The *vagina* is the canal inside the body that extends upward from the vaginal opening.

At the closed end of the vagina sits the *cervix*, a round, firm donut-shaped structure that makes up the lowest end of the uterus. For some women, the cervix is fairly close to the vaginal opening, while for others, it's so deep inside that it can't be felt with an inserted finger. The entire uterus is designed to move. It contracts and relaxes during the menstrual cycle (who hasn't felt menstrual cramps?) and provides a home for a growing fetus during pregnancy. Some women find it quite pleasurable to have their cervix stimulated through sexual penetration, while for others it is uncomfortable. When everything is functioning properly and the uterus is mobile, that type of penetration is nice; however, if the mobility is not what it should be, the same stimulation can cause discomfort or even pain.

In our discussion of exterior anatomy, we mentioned that the clitoris is actually much bigger than the clitoral glans. Remember, the glans is the only exterior part of the clitoris. The rest of it is internal. How much more is there? Here, we'll show you:

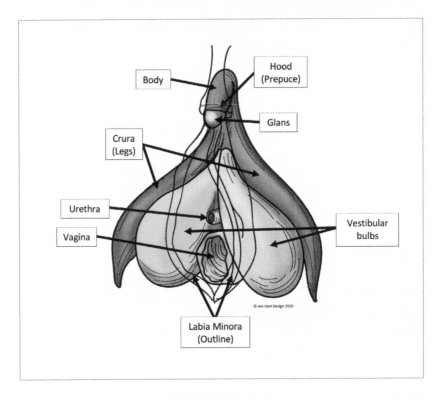

That much more

Anatomists only learned the full extent of the clitoris in 1998.[8] What's with that? How could something so amazing have been overlooked for so long? Here's the best news about the clitoris: its only function is to give us pleasure. As you can see in the image above, the clitoral glans is at the end of the clitoral shaft. The other end of the clitoral shaft splits twice to form the two *crura* or "legs" of the clitoris and the *vestibular bulb* each one has at its end. These bulbs continue through and behind the labia and extend down toward the anus on either side of the urethra and vaginal canal. The entire clitoral structure contains erectile tissue that swells up with blood during sexual arousal.

There's an important bit of the arousal network that isn't pictured in this image: the *G-spot*. That's because, as of this writing, the G-spot has not been scientifically proven to exist. From Elizabeth's vantage point, it exists; after all, women have been sharing secrets of the G-spot for centuries! But from Dee's point of view, the actual science around it is inconclusive. Some studies have found a G-spot, while others have not, so we cannot say with certainty that it's there. We're not the only ones confused by this. A piece published by *Cosmopolitan* magazine suggested that women's pleasure advocates were quick to jump on anecdotal evidence of a G-spot, or at least a generalized G-spot-related area. Yet the science hasn't come through to back that up. And worse, many women have felt pressured to find their G-spot and inadequate when they couldn't. So in the end, *Cosmo* decided to throw in the towel and say, at least for now, there is no anatomical G-spot.[9] Even though we're split, we appreciate their rationale! We certainly don't want any discussion in this book to make any woman feel like they're incomplete.

That said, anecdotally, many women talk about experiencing significant pleasure in this region, and their stories often align with each other. And who are we to deny any woman her pleasure? Therefore, in this book, we will treat the G-spot as if it does exist because doing so might bring you more pleasure, and that's our whole goal. Due to differences in body shape and size, the exact location of the G-spot varies from woman to woman, and some women feel they do not have one at all. Of the women who report having a G-spot, they generally note that it can be found on the anterior (front) vaginal wall, that the tissue covering it is spongy and somewhat ridged, and that it swells with adequate arousal, making it easier to feel with an inserted finger once they're turned on. Sometimes, stimulating this area can create what's called *female ejaculate*. We'll discuss this more in Chapter Seven.

Also located inside and helping to hold most of these parts in place is a complex network of *pelvic floor muscles*. This is a group of muscles inside the pelvis that run from the front (starting near the pubic bone) all the way to the back (ending at the tailbone). Here's a very simplified image of what is, in fact, a very complex set of muscles:

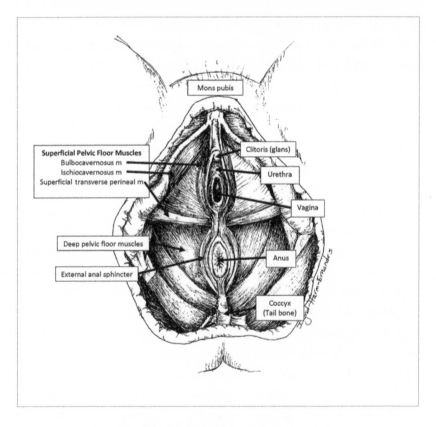

Look at all of those! And these are just the main ones.
Women—we're so complex!

The pelvic floor muscles provide support to hold the organs in your pelvis—such as your bladder, urethra, uterus, and rectum—in place.

Beyond that, they provide overall support as a part of your core. The pelvic floor muscles also help you control your urine and stool, which is a pretty big deal, and they do one more crucial thing: provide the delightful pulsating pleasure that happens with orgasm.

The pelvic floor muscles are very important, and they deserve your utmost attention and care! They can be affected by all sorts of things—like childbirth, menopause, chronic respiratory illness, surgery, and trauma—and it's not unusual for women to need help conditioning or reconditioning them. They can be too weak or, commonly, far too tight for the arousal network to function properly. In fact, we know that excessive tension in the pelvic floor muscles, a focus of Dee's clinical treatment approach, can be responsible for a whole lot of women's sexual pain. Anecdotally, Elizabeth's clients have reported that arousal and pleasure can actually decrease some of that abnormal tension, suggesting that pleasure and pain impact one another. Whether that could prove true for you or not, we think the pelvic floor muscles are important enough that we've given them a lot of attention in this book.

Okay, so we've covered your outsides and your insides, showing you the main parts of your arousal network and briefly discussing how it all works. But anatomy is not one-size-fits-all. It's true that Jaime didn't know how most of her arousal network was designed to work. But Elizabeth sensed something even more troubling: Jamie had never been that interested in her arousal network because, deep down, she thought her vulva was *ugly and weird*. She feared that something was *wrong with her*. No one had ever told Jaime that her anatomy was more than likely *normal*.

What Is "Normal," Anyway?

This section is near and dear to our hearts because we've heard far too often how deeply ashamed women are of their bodies. This shame often includes *low genital self-esteem*, which is dissatisfaction with the appearance of one's genitals. When they tell us about their shame, it's painful both personally and professionally to hear. That's because in almost fifty years of combined professional work in this field, *we've never seen an ugly vulva.*

Most women have a very narrow view of what "normal" vulvas look like, thanks in part to the textbook vulva we showed you before. And many have no reference for what vulvas should smell or taste like, except a vague sense that they should smell and taste "normal," too, whatever that may be. But there's a real lack of education around what "normal" truly is, and it's causing a lot of damage. Women who are worried about what their vulvas look like, smell like, and taste like have a harder time experiencing pleasure.

There's research to prove it: studies have shown that there is a correlation between genital self-esteem and better sex. A positive genital self-image is associated with higher arousal, lubrication, orgasm, satisfaction, and an absence of pain.[10] Additionally, those who have a positive genital self-image feel more sexually attractive.[11] Studies also show that having a negative genital self-image may decrease sexual satisfaction as well as women's motivation to avoid risky sexual behavior.[12]

It's not just the textbook vulva that has women confused; porn is a huge part of the problem too. As with other sorts of media, porn—be it in print or on video—has increasingly skewed public opinion of what is normal and beautiful. Images of vulvas that don't conform to a cultural, standardized norm of beauty are digitally altered to enhance color and change their shape and size. That's right: vulva Photoshop. Another factor influencing public perspectives is that porn stars and models are often hired, in part, based on the petite size and shape of their vulvas, which is not representative of the average woman. This means the viewing audience never sees the true genital variety in terms of size, shape, and color. Like it or not, the media, especially porn, has negatively impacted how women see their bodies and has put undue societal pressures upon women to look a certain way.

newsflash: this isn't new information. In 1933, Robert Latou Dickinson, MD, FACS, published a book called *Human Sex Anatomy*. We love this book! It includes a set of absolutely gorgeous, hand-drawn images of vulvas, each of which is unique and special and different. Here are a few of our favorites:

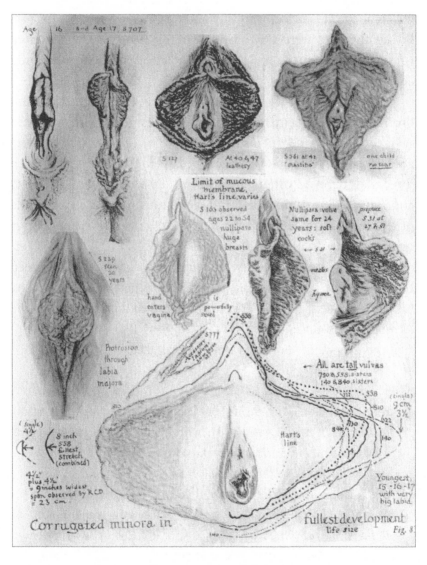

They are all magnificent!

It's amazing that these were published in 1933, but it's also really sad. These beautiful drawings appear to have gone unnoticed in the medical literature from that point on. Nowadays, most medical textbooks don't include diversity like this; instead, they just show that same textbook vulva with its tidy pubic hair (or no hair at all), small, symmetrical lips, and rosy shade of pink. Each one of the vulvas above are perfectly normal and healthy—and unlike the textbook vulva, they were drawn while looking at the vulvas of different women. (To see more images like this, check out vulvalove.com/additional-resources.)

Vulvas aren't the only things that are diverse; vaginas are diverse too. They vary in length. As we mentioned before, some can be short, with the cervix just a knuckle or two inside, while others are longer such that you will never be able to touch the cervix with fingers alone. And others are somewhere in between. Diversity continues: some vaginal openings are quite tight and small, while others have an opening that's, well, more open. This can change over time due to hormonal changes, increased or decreased tension in the pelvic floor muscles, uterine prolapse, arousal (keep reading; we've got a lot more to say about that!), and more. The take-home message for you is that *vaginas and their openings are as diverse as people.*

And every single one of them is normal.

A Note from Dee:

Your ability to fit things inside your vagina is not only determined by its size. That's because your vagina doesn't live alone; it has a lot of neighbors, and those neighbors can sometimes get fussy.

We'll start with the viscera, or organs. Think of the vulva like a clock—the clitoris is at 12:00 and the anus is at 6:00. At 12:00, or sitting right above the vagina when lying down, is the urethra, which leads up to the bladder. Then there's the cervix, which is the lowest portion of the uterus, hanging at the top end of the vagina, between the bladder and the

rectum. Below the vagina, or at 6:00, you'll find the anus. The
pelvic floor muscles support these organs, as does the fascia,
or connective tissue.

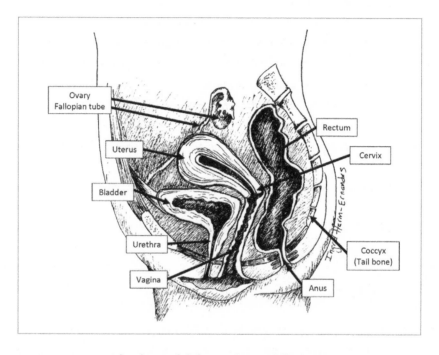

It's a beautiful day in the neighborhood.

So what this all means is that issues with any of these things
can affect how it feels when things go inside of your vagina.
For instance, if you're constipated—meaning your rectum
is full of hard, compacted stool—it decreases the space that
you have for intercourse, which may not be very comfortable
and can diminish your pleasure. If you have an irritable
bladder that gets bumped while having sex, it can cause
pain during and after the experience. You may feel like
you have an infection (UTI), but most of the time, it's just
post-penetration irritation. For women who have a history
of endometriosis, when the tissue that is supposed to grow
on the inside of the uterus grows on the outside too, having

something jostle the uterus can be really painful. The uterus is supposed to get out of the way with penetration, but the extra tissue often prevents that from happening. There are also five small hip rotator muscles next to the vaginal wall, so if the hip muscles are tight, they can cause problems too.

And that's only a short list! There are all sorts of things around and connected to your vagina that can limit what feels good. This is important for women to know because it's not always your vagina that's causing pain; sometimes, it's the neighbors!

Understanding diversity helps us to realize that there is no one "normal" vulva or vagina—they're *all* normal! So now, we're going to introduce you to your own, starting with your vulva.

Prescription 1

Introduction to Your Vulva

This is the first prescription that Elizabeth gave to Jaime, and the first one we're giving to you. You're going to be looking at your vulva. Many women have never done anything like this before. And even if you have, looking again can be useful. When Elizabeth asked one of her clients if she knew what her vulva looked like, her response was, "Well, I don't think I could pick it out of a line-up, if that's what you're asking!" By the end of this prescription, we want you to be able to pick your vulva out of a line-up; we want you to know what it looks like and feels like, without a doubt. Repeat this prescription to strengthen your genital self-esteem, reminding yourself every time that your vulva is beautiful, unique, and special.

Not only that, this prescription can have major health benefits. That's because when you know what's "normal" for your unique anatomy, it's much easier to determine when something is off. With vulvar and other cancers of the sexual organs on the rise,[13] it's really important for every woman to have awareness of her genital health. Notice what type of discharge your vagina produces, which may change in consistency and increase in volume at midcycle—if you're still menstruating—and what colors, smells, and consistencies are normal for you. Pay attention to the color and shape of your labia so you can quickly spot any abnormal growths. Take notice of any unusual itching, bleeding, or tearing that doesn't go away. This attention allows you spot any changes, which in turn should prompt you to seek out medical help more quickly.

Before you get started, we should note that some women might experience minor pain or burning as they do this. If this doesn't happen, disregard this paragraph. But if it does, we encourage you to touch yourself very gently and pay very close attention to your breath. We'll talk a lot more about pain and the breath in Chapter Two. But for now, just take a few deep breaths before moving forward. This will help you to relax as you gently explore your vulva. If you still have discomfort, pain, or burning after a few minutes of deep breathing, you can use an ice pack to alleviate it. Be sure to cover the ice pack with a towel so it is not directly on your vulva, and leave it there for no more than twenty minutes at a time.

What You'll Need:

- At least fifteen minutes of complete privacy.

- A mirror—if possible, one that magnifies.

- Good overall lighting and, if possible, a flashlight or flashlight app.

- A journal and a pen.

Let's Get Started!

- Arrange yourself comfortably on the floor, a bed, couch, or armchair. Prop your back, legs, etc. up with pillows if needed. Make sure you're warm; relaxation is key here, so get comfortable. You'll be seated like this for a while.

- Get naked from the waist down (except socks, if you like them!) and spread your legs.

- Place the mirror between your thighs and close enough for you to see. Adjust it so you can see your entire vulva. Use the flashlight if you need to.

- Breathe. And again. Keep breathing.

- Start by taking in everything you see. Begin to notice the shape, size, and color of all the parts of your vulva. Identify the clitoral glans, clitoral hood, inner and outer labia, urethra, and vaginal opening. Pay attention to the sensations you feel as you do this.

- As you do so, notice any feelings that come up. Jot them down in your notebook without judgment; simply write down what you experience.

- Notice your breath again. Are you breathing deeply? If you're not, pause and return to your breath before continuing.

- When you're ready, take a look at your outer labia and notice how that feels.

- Then, gently spread your labia. Notice how that feels too.

- Pause to write down what you noticed. Do so without judgment—remember, all vulvas are beautiful! In addition to the sensations, you may also want to write down any emotions that come to the surface.

- Look at the opening of your vagina. Gently place your thumb at the bottom of the vaginal opening, just above the anus, with the tip pointing inside of the vagina. This is still the vulva; it doesn't become the vagina until you get inside. It's also the area where most women who feel pain notice their pain beginning to spike. Apply gentle pressure to this area and notice what happens. Does it feel good? Does it feel painful? If it hurts, does that pain feel familiar? Write it down, describing the pain in detail (burning, aching, stabbing, pins and needles, etc.) along with what you were doing when you felt it before.

- Check in with your breathing once again and return to deep breaths if you find yourself holding your breath or breathing quickly.

- Now find your clitoral hood and gently lift it back, as much as you can comfortably, to expose your clitoral glans. Does your hood move easily? Can you see your glans? How far under the hood is it? How does it feel to lift the hood like this? If you can touch your glans, what does that feel like? A number of women have a pasty, white substance called *smegma* under the hood or between the outer and inner labia. This is a normal substance that helps with lubrication. Don't worry, it doesn't mean you're not keeping yourself clean.

- Release the hood and put your finger on top of it. Gently roll your finger back and forth to feel the roundness of the clitoral shaft underneath. Notice how this feels. Pause and write it down.

- Again, check in with your breath, being sure to inhale deeply and exhale completely.

- With a different finger, find your perineal body and your anus. Gently touch this area, noticing any sensations, and write them down. Also notice any emotions that arise and write those down too. (As you continue to explore your vulva, be sure to not use this finger again until you've washed it thoroughly. There are normal bacteria hanging around the area, and washing your finger will prevent you from accidentally spreading it where it doesn't belong.)

- Remove your hand and study your vulva once again. Has the color changed? That is a natural reaction. Did you experience any change in sensation? That's normal too. Make note of any changes. Write down any emotions or memories that came up during the exercise.

- When you've finished, cup one hand over the top of your pubic bone with your fingers pointed downward toward your anus and let your head rest back on a pillow. While in this position, relax and breathe deeply for another few minutes.

- Release your hand slowly and close your legs. You can put your clothes back on if that would make you more comfortable as you complete the prescription.

- To finish the prescription, sit or lie comfortably with your eyes shut to let the experience land in your body. Breathe normally. Get up when you feel ready.

- If there are any last things you want to write down, do so now. You may also notice sensations or emotions after the prescription is complete. You may find yourself remembering events or comments that negatively affected your genital self-esteem. Writing them down will be very useful for you, and we encourage you to do so!

(Vulvar) Knowledge Is Power!

With that, we congratulate you for finishing your first prescription! It's a big step in the direction of your own pleasure, and we know that it may not have been easy or comfortable. For Jaime, completing Prescription 1 was challenging, but she stuck with it and felt better about her vulva afterward.

This chapter offered you a strong—and hopefully, pleasurable—primer on the female arousal network. With our guidance, you began to explore the anatomy that helps you feel sexual pleasure. We discussed the vast diversity of genital appearance and introduced the importance of genital self-esteem, which can have a huge effect on our ability to feel pleasure. And then, you took the plunge to explore your own unique, beautiful, normal vulva!

You learned that when we don't understand or accept our bodies, our access to pleasure is limited, even though unlimited pleasure is exactly what our bodies were designed to experience. But there are other things that can impact our ability to access pleasurable experiences too. One of these things is pain. In the next chapter, we'll explore pain more deeply, getting into the details of genital and sexual pain, why some women have it, and what women can do to reduce it.

CHAPTER TWO

Understanding Your Pain

A Note from Dee:

Susana was twenty-one. Her doctor sent her to me because she was having pain with sex. She told me that the first time she had sex, as a teenager, she didn't know what to expect— she had heard that it would hurt, but she didn't expect it to hurt as much as it did. She described being in pain for the next three days, and that her pain intensified when she walked, went to the bathroom, or sat in a chair. Sex wasn't so bad anymore, she explained to me, but it still hurt every time. I asked her some basic questions, such as whether she was ever bothered just by wearing underwear (yes; she felt a burning sometimes, which the friction from the underwear intensified) or put in a tampon (definitely; she didn't use tampons because the process of getting them in and out was just too painful).

We began discussing her childhood. As a child, Susana frequently suffered from urinary tract infections that were treated with urethral dilation. She told me she hated going to the doctor and sometimes wouldn't share her symptoms with her mother to avoid going back to the doctor's office. It was both scary and humiliating. I could feel her discomfort as we discussed these issues. I asked her how many other doctors she had seen prior to the one who referred her to me; there were four. The first three, she explained, told her that she just needed to relax before having sex. One gave her a prescription for lidocaine, telling her to use it on the vulva before having sex. She never filled it. I could only imagine that seeing all of these doctors was very difficult for Susana, and that it must have been awful when, time after time, doing so didn't resolve her pain. When she wasn't answering my questions, Susana looked at the floor. I felt terrible for her. I really wanted to give her a big hug and tell her that I understood.

Finally, Susana disclosed the reason she had been so desperately seeking help recently, even though these issues had gone on for years: she was in love with a new boyfriend, and she really wanted to enjoy sex with him. She had hoped that her feelings for him would make their first sexual encounter magical. But that didn't happen; it still hurt. Embarrassed, Susana tried to hide the pain, but he had seen it in her face. He encouraged her to talk about it, and for the first time, she discussed her pain openly with a partner. Her boyfriend responded by saying that he didn't want to have sex if it hurt her. With his support, she went from doctor to doctor in search of a solution. Finally, she found the doctor who sent her to me to see if physical therapy could help.

I cannot tell you how many Susanas have been in my office. She needed compassionate, comprehensive medical care, and practitioners who truly valued her ability to access sexual pleasure. If Susana's story sounds familiar, then this chapter is for you.

Many women experience vulvar pain, pelvic pain, and pain with sex. As many as twenty-five million women in the United States have had pain or burning at the opening of the vagina (which is considered part of the vulva) at some point in their lives.[14] When doing an informal study of the women coming to our VulvaLove workshops and talks, we were shocked and surprised to learn that they too experienced pain with sex. Note that the women in our community are sex-positive, have received a pleasure-forward education, and are, generally speaking, more open than most when talking about sex. Yet a whopping eighteen out of twenty-four (74 percent) of our unpublished survey respondents noted that they had experienced pain with sex at some point in their lives.

After years of silence, the media is starting to give these unfortunate truths some traction. Recent articles in *InStyle*[15] and *The Week*[16] have addressed the pain many women have with sex, and the comments sections and shares of these articles demonstrate just how many women have been waiting to see their experience represented in print. The American College of Obstetricians and Gynecologists now has statistics on their website showing that 75 percent of women have had pain with sex[17]—a much more scientific number that directly mirrors our informal VulvaLove findings. Women who experience pain find relief just hearing this statistic. It speaks directly to what they have long felt: sex hurts.

This chapter is about genital pain: how it's diagnosed by the medical world, how pain is perceived, and what you can do to make it better. We believe that women like Susana deserve the help that they are looking for—and that women who are too ashamed, too embarrassed, or simply unaware that pain-free sex is possible find solutions too. Here's the truth: Your vulva and vagina shouldn't hurt, nor should sex be painful (unless, of course, that's your kink). Inserting tampons and having routine gynecological exams shouldn't hurt at the opening of your vagina, either. If everything is going as it's supposed to, your vulva and vagina should bring you pleasure and joy, not pain and discomfort. (Well, gynecological exams and tampons may not be too joyful, but you get what we're talking about.)

So, let's talk about pain, because when you get down to it, there are a lot of ways that women describe how their vulvas and vaginas hurt. When it comes to pain at the vulva, the most common descriptors women use are *burning, itching, hot, stabbing,* and *aching.* Women also describe their vulvas as feeling *tight, stinging, tingling,* and *pricking,* and they describe the pain itself as *heavy, pressing, crushing, sharp, hurting, squeezing,* and *tearing.*[18] These words all describe a sort of discomfort that we're lumping into *pain.* We want to be clear about that because, while some women are fully aware that they are in pain, others use another word (or words) for it—but if the word is any of those listed above, for our intents and purposes, it's pain.

Other women may not have vulvar pain with insertion but do have pain once things are inside the vagina—like fingers, tampons, toys, and penises. As we described in the last chapter, your vagina has neighbors, and there are certain situations wherein things can bump up against something that doesn't feel so good. But if there is significant, ongoing, chronic pain with insertion, something else is likely going on.

As you explore your relationship with pain, it may be very useful to rate your pain on a scale from 0–10 on a regular basis. Watch how it changes over time, using the scale to help you track. We'll use this scale later in the book too.

Pain Scale

No Pain

0 – Pain free.

Mild Pain
Nagging, annoying but doesn't really interfere with daily activities.

1 – Pain is very mild, barely noticeable. Most of the time you don't think about it.
2 – Minor pain. Annoying and may have occasional stronger twinges.
3 – Pain is noticeable and distracting; however, you can get used to it and adapt.

Moderate Pain
Interferes significantly with daily activities.

4 – Moderate pain. If you were deeply involved in an activity, it can be ignored for a period of time but is still distracting.
5 – Moderately strong pain. It can't be ignored for more than a few minutes, but with effort you still can manage to work or participate in some social activities.
6 – Moderately strong pain that interferes with normal daily activities. Difficulty concentrating.

Severe Pain
Disabling; unable to perform daily activities.

7 – Severe pain that dominates your senses and significantly limits your ability to perform normal daily activities or maintain social relationships. Interferes with sleep.
8 – Intense pain. Physical activity is severely limited. Conversing requires great effort.
9 – Excruciating pain. Unable to converse. Crying out and/or moaning uncontrollably.
10 – Unspeakable pain. Bedridden and possibly delirious. Very few people will ever experience this level of pain.

Pain Scale[19]

A Note from Dee:

The medical community doesn't do a great job of accurately identifying the types of pain women have with sex. I'll introduce a few terms that you may have heard. These terms will help you better understand what your health practitioners may label your diagnosis.

If you have been experiencing pain in your vulva, par-

ticularly at the opening of your vagina, it may be diagnosed as vulvodynia. Vulvodynia *is defined as pain in the vulva that has lasted longer than three months and that has no other identifiable cause or disease. The percentage of women in the US who experience vulvodynia ranges from 9 to 18 percent,*[20] *which works out to anywhere from fifteen to thirty million women. The pain can be unremitting and felt throughout the vulva* (spontaneous vulvodynia) *or felt only when anything comes in contact with the opening of the vagina* (provoked vestibulodynia, *also called* PVD). *Currently, researchers don't know what causes vulvodynia but know it's not a result of infection, cancer, nerve disorders, trauma, lack of estrogen, or from skin disease. They do think, however, that there can be predisposing factors contributing to the pain, like genetic disorders, sensitivity to certain foods, or pelvic floor muscle spasm.*[21] *This vexing pain syndrome has stymied medical researchers and practitioners since it was first studied in the 1980s.*

There is no real word to categorize pain that comes with deep thrusting or putting something else, like a tampon, deep inside your vagina. General aching or cramping in your pelvic region is called pelvic pain, *and sometimes pain with sex is just called, well,* pain with sex.

There are two additional diagnoses that you might also have heard. First, dyspareunia *is a term that refers to any unwanted pain with sex. It is a vague diagnosis, as it does nothing to describe the type of pain or where it's located. Dyspareunia can be caused by any number of things like lack of arousal, chronic urinary tract infections, skin disorders, or endometriosis.*

Another common diagnosis is vaginismus. *Women with vaginismus may experience extreme fear and avoidance associated with genital touch or impending genital touch, whether sexual or not. That fear can cause overactive pelvic floor muscle tension and may or may not cause vulvar pain. Unfortunately, for diagnostic purposes, vaginismus is classified as a psychological disorder, not a physical one. It is a source of great emotional pain and shame and deserves proper treatment. But this diagnosis is significant because, for some women, receiving this label means their psychological symptoms get all the attention while their physical pain is left untreated.*

Any pain that persists or recurs for more than three months, anywhere in the body, is considered chronic. Therefore, regardless of whether you experience pain all the time or only with certain activities (e.g., sex), if you've struggled with it for at least ninety days, it may also be classified as chronic vaginal pain or chronic vulvar pain.

The reason I've spent so much time on these terms is that these diagnoses can be confusing. Pain, no matter how you label it, all too often stops women from engaging in any type of sexual behavior, whether solo or partnered, robbing them of pleasure. Understanding how your medical practitioners view and categorize your pain may help you advocate for yourself in the exam room.

We know that as many as three in every four women of reproductive age experience pain with sex.[22] We also know that the effects of this pain go far beyond the physical symptoms; it can affect women's ability to connect and be intimate with their partner, which brings a host of other issues, including dissociation, depression, shame, and guilt. In our personal experience, we have heard many women blame themselves for the pain they experience—perhaps they are concerned that they touched themselves too much as a child, or that traumatic sexual experiences "broke" them, that they had sex that was somehow immoral, or that they used tampons too early. Hearing these fears and theories is heartbreaking to us.

Women have come to both of our offices speaking of pain, and we know that many more suffer in silence, never seeking help. Sixty percent of the women who do seek help visit three to four doctors *on average* before receiving a diagnosis, and even then, only 40 percent of those receive the right diagnosis.[23]

Many doctors simply don't know what to do to help a woman who presents with such pain. In today's healthcare system, medical practitioners haven't received adequate training on how to talk to their patients about genital health, function, and sex.[24] You might be surprised to learn that only clinicians with a specific interest in women's sexual health have received trainings in how to talk about sex and sexual matters with their patients. It's not that doctors are withholding information—they just aren't resourced with that specific knowledge or skill. They certainly didn't learn it during medical school, which we think is a major oversight in the medical field.

All too often, women with pain are told by their healthcare providers to "just relax." Now, let's be clear: relaxation is a big part of it, and this chapter will explain how that works in depth. That said, we think that "just relax" can be a really condescending, dismissive thing to say to a woman. How do you "just relax" when you don't know you're tense in the first place?

Over the years, Dee has watched with concern as more and more practitioners address chronic vulvar pain by prescribing numbing creams like lidocaine for use directly on the vulva and vaginal opening before sex. (*"What?!"* Elizabeth just spit out her tea.) Even more shocking is that many physicians and some physical therapists opt to numb the vulva with lidocaine prior to internal exams and/or physical therapy treatment. While numbing the vulva temporarily reduces genital pain, it encourages women to ignore their pain threshold, whether it be during an internal exam or treatment or penetrative sex. Deadening the sensitivity at the vulva might allow an otherwise impossible internal exam, but it is not a long-term solution to genital pain. It doesn't fix the problem, and it reduces women's access to the pleasure they deserve.

If you have been experiencing pain with sex, or vulvar/vaginal pain in general, please know that we hear you and that you are not alone. We'll explain how pain works and go over some of the most common culprits that cause it. Then, we'll look at how reducing tension and opening to pleasure may help lower the levels of pain you experience, or even eradicate it completely.

How Pain Works

Our brains are filled with neurons. Part of their job is to tell us how to react to things. When we are presented with any sort of stimulus, our neurons fire naturally occurring chemicals called *neurotransmitters*. After the same neurons fire the same neurotransmitters a few times, they create patterns called *neural pathways*. Once a neural pathway is created, it's far easier to follow the existing pathway than to rewrite it—much like how in the jungle, it's far easier to follow the path you already walked and cut with a machete than it is to create a new path altogether. In fact, the more we travel the same path, the easier it becomes to travel, and the harder, comparatively, it becomes to create a new one.

From a neural standpoint, pain has an evolutionary purpose: it is meant to warn you that you either are hurting or are about to hurt yourself. In other words, it arouses you to current or impending danger. But this system can get confused and misfire, either overestimating the danger or indicating that there is danger when, in fact, there is none. What this means is that the experience of pain is not always reliable in assessing how hurt we actually are. Sometimes, we're just used to firing the same set of neurons in the same pattern. Our brains have formed a habit that it repeats over and over again, causing extreme pain that serves no evolutionary function.

This is a delicate subject; we by no means want to suggest that your pain isn't real. It's absolutely real! And in some cases, it's indicating that you *are* doing damage to your body somehow—which is why we always suggest that you look for a doctor who can help. But if doctor after doctor can't find the source of your pain, it may be worth exploring whether your brain is signaling pain disproportionately.

Because if this is the case, we have good news: old habits can be changed. Just like you can train yourself to remember to take a pill or supplement before breakfast, or to stretch before going for a run, you can train your brain to fire in ways that are healthier and more pleasant for your daily experience. It's not necessarily easy—just ask someone who has stopped a really tough habit, like swearing or biting their fingernails. Creating new neural pathways is no small task. But science shows us that it is possible.

This concept is called *neuroplasticity*. Essentially, the theory around neuroplasticity states that the brain is able to create new neural connections. Those new connections form new neural pathways (new paths in the jungle), which become easier and easier to follow the more often we use them. As these new pathways become habitual, they can allow you to rewire significant portions of your neural network. Not only that, but in some cases, the brain can actually create new neurons in a process called *neurogenesis*. The science around neuroplasticity is emerging rapidly and is very exciting, especially for people who experience chronic pain. It suggests that *even when we can't get rid of what's causing the pain, we can change how we experience that pain.*[25]

It's also important to understand how the body and brain respond to pain. Interestingly, from a neurochemical standpoint, the response to pain is very similar to the response to pleasure. When you experience pain, your brain begins to release endogenous opioids, like *beta-endorphins* and *enkephalins*, into specific, pain-related brain regions and from the pituitary gland into the body. These endogenous opioids act like morphine to block pain transmission, eventually dulling the painful stimulus, allowing you to tolerate it if you cannot avoid it. And the brain learns from that experience to anticipate when pain might occur next so you can avoid it next time *before* it happens. That anticipation is driven in large part by two other neurotransmitters, *dopamine* and *noradrenaline*. When a particular context or certain stimuli in the environment arouse a memory of pain, noradrenaline is activated to induce a general arousal state of alarm, and dopamine is activated to enable your brain to attend to the stimuli so that your body can make immediate avoidance responses. This is very similar to their role in pleasure, where opioids are activated and generate a pleasurable state, which then sensitizes noradrenaline and dopamine so that you can focus on the pleasure. And the states of pain and pleasure interact. Think runner's high after completing a grueling marathon. This may help explain how the threat of pain in the context of bondage/ discipline or dominance/sadism or submission/masochism, commonly known as BDSM, can also become sexually arousing if it is connected to sexual pleasure.

We know that certain types of sexually specific stimulation can alleviate pain too. The G-spot is one such example. In the last chapter, we discussed that the jury is still out on the existence of the G-spot. Studies that support its presence report that simulating the G-spot may actually alleviate the experience of pain. It's important to understand the difference between an anesthetic (which reduces sensation overall) and an analgesic (which reduces pain while keeping all other sensations intact). The studies show that while G-spot stimulation is not anesthetic, it is analgesic—which means it can reduce pain even as pleasure increases.[26] In fact, this can happen with all forms of pleasure. Studies have shown that any sort of pleasurable stimuli, including sex and the enjoyment of food, can trigger the release of pain-reducing neurotransmitters like opioids into key areas of the brain.

So, we can see that in many cases, treating pain with pleasure is effective in the short term. But what might happen if we repeatedly use pleasure to reduce pain? Could neuroplasticity and neurogenesis actually help us rewire the brain into a pattern of pleasure and out of a pattern of pain?

It's an interesting question, and one that much of this book is dedicated to exploring. But some types of sexual pain are easily preventable, circumventing the need for a brain-rewire. Sometimes, the cause of sexual pain can be easily assessed and eradicated. This next section takes a look at some of the most common examples.

Common, Nonmedical Causes of Sexual Pain

Two other common causes of pain are inadequate lubrication and insufficient arousal.

Far too often, when our clients and patients come in telling us how sex hurts, we quickly find out that they aren't producing enough lubrication for sex to feel good. Look, sex is all about body parts rubbing together. That friction is a huge part of what helps sex feel good. At the same time, too much friction without enough lubrication can make sex feel really bad. Our bodies produce natural lubrication as our arousal increases; however, some women produce a lot and some not enough. For those in the latter group, adding lube from a tube can make sex feel a whole lot better.

Some women need lube for most, if not all, sexual encounters. They tend to run hot and dry. These women have lube stored by their bedside, in the kitchen messy drawer; they stash it in their purses and even in their car. Then there are others who don't need extra lube at all. It's about different body chemistries and different hormonal makeups. There is nothing wrong with using lube. If you need it, lube makes sex a whole lot better, a whole lot of the time! It's relatively inexpensive, easy to find, and a little bit lasts a long time. We'll talk more about what type of lube to look for in the prescriptions, but let this be the first (of many) public service announcements you'll find in this book about the wonders of good lube. There's no shame in needing lube. We know that the ability to self-lubricate is related to our hormones, and some women just don't produce that much on their own (if you're postmenopausal, you'll know exactly what we're talking about!). And it doesn't necessarily mean that you aren't enjoying the sexual activity you're engaged in.

At the same time, we cannot overlook one of the main reasons we believe women have a need for lube: inadequate arousal. That's why we say—*if you're not reaching full arousal, the need for lube is only part of the problem.*

See, the truth is that many women are having penetrative sex before their bodies are ready for it. Let's face it: it takes women longer to reach full arousal than it does men.

A Note from Elizabeth:

If there were one phrase I wish I could say I coined, it's pre-mature penetration. Mull that over for a few seconds. Let it roll through your body. The concept of premature penetration is about timing, suggesting that if anything has been inserted into a woman's vagina before she is highly aroused, she's been prematurely penetrated. Many practitioners use the phrase; however, I must give credit to first hearing it from my fellow sex educator, Sheri Winston.[27]

All too often, women succumb to vaginal penetration before they're ready. There are a lot of reasons why this happens. One of them can be feeling pressured by a partner to have sex when you don't want to. Too many women just "go for it" or "put up with it" to please their partner. Another reason is that a lot of women simply don't feel much or ever reach an adequate state of arousal. There's a huge difference between what it feels like to be penetrated prematurely and the feeling that comes with penetration after we're highly aroused, fully engorged, and completely turned on. The bottom line is: if something's inside your vagina and it doesn't feel good, you were penetrated before your body was ready.

But what about a quickie, you ask? A lot of us have had them. Sometimes a quickie is fulfilling. The caveat here is that the woman is the driver and open to the quickie; she feels desire for sex and wants to be penetrated. Here's where having a good lube by your bedside comes in handy. In that case, being prematurely penetrated when you are not fully physically aroused is your choice. Having the occasional

quickie as part of your overall sexual repertoire is okay by us,
as long as it is not your only lovemaking experience and it
doesn't cause pain. If you experience premature penetration,
I suggest that you take the time to learn and feel your full
arousal before having another quickie.

My deepest wish is that every woman waits until her
mind, body, vulva, and vagina are fully aroused before she
is penetrated. Full stop.

You've probably heard people say that "size doesn't matter." And perhaps you have found that to be true—or not. Some women have come to us reporting that their partner's penises are uncomfortably big, while others have mentioned that they wish their partner were, well, more endowed.

Here, again, is where arousal plays an important role. When a woman is aroused, her vaginal opening can accommodate a variety of sizes in terms of girth (diameter), and her vagina can be equally hospitable with regard to different penile lengths.[28] There are times, however, when deep thrusting can hurt even if a woman is fully aroused, but the problem isn't her vaginal tissue. When the cervix takes the brunt of deep thrusting and the uterus isn't mobile, pain is often the result. Changing the angle of penetration can help, as can adding products designed to restrict the depth of penetration, which can be found at many sex shops or online.

But regardless of the type of pain, a lot of sexual pain begins with tension in the pelvic floor muscles. Furthermore, this creates a cycle, as increased pain yields increased tension. Let's explore how that cycle works.

The Role of Tension

As we presented earlier in this chapter, tension is a tricky subject because we know that many women have been told that the pain is all in their head, and they need to just relax or have a glass of wine and sex won't hurt. This is an overly simplistic and often callous assertion and one we don't want to repeat. At the same time, tension *does* often play a role in pain—and, unfortunately, it isn't always addressed. Once tension is recognized, however, you can work to reduce it.

On a physical level, tension in the pelvic floor muscles can decrease the size of the vaginal opening, which can cause pain with penetration. Most women have no idea that this tension exists inside their bodies. They just know that when anything is inserted into their vagina, it hurts. Most women experiencing painful sex are physically unable to actively relax their pelvic floor muscles. Their first step is to regain control of their muscles. Just as flexing a muscle takes practice, relaxing it can take practice too. Women should be able to fully squeeze and let go of their pelvic floor muscles at will. Those who do not have this control over their muscles will often experience pain with sex.

Women who have pain with sex or chronic vulvar pain often have tension throughout their bodies, especially in their hips and lower backs. Relief from this tension can often be reduced through stretching. And believe it or not, for many of our clients and patients, adding simple stretching exercises to their daily routine to address the hips, lower back, and pelvic region has made a huge difference in their pelvic floor muscle function—and, consequently, their pain.

Holding tension also affects the breath. Breathing, one of our most basic functions, is often not as effective as it should be, especially for people who have a history of anxiety, chronic pain, depression, or painful sex. Proper breathing, which we'll describe in the prescription, can help to calm your anxiety, slow your heart rate, and relax tension throughout your body.

Even when there are other causes for pain, tension can make it a whole lot worse. Furthermore, pain itself is often the root cause of tension—just as tension can also be the root cause of pain. Regardless of where it starts, pain and tension together create an amplifying cycle that is hard to break. We tense up, we feel pain, and then we tense up more. As you learned earlier in the chapter, physical responses are often associated with our neural pathways. That means that this cycle can become a habit not only in our brains, but also in our bodies. Now we have the brain telling the body to tense in anticipation of pain, and the body tensing in response, causing even more pain. This is called *reflexive splinting*. Once it's ingrained as a pattern, it can be hard to break.

Our brains are designed to help our bodies do amazing things. This is why it's also important to understand what's happening in the brain when there's tension during sex. If you don't know how mental tension works—or, specifically, how it connects to your sexuality—you may not be aware of the impact it can have on your body, your arousal, or your intimacy.

Our nervous system is wired to protect us from anything threatening. When faced with danger, how we process and react to the situation is important, as it could be a matter of life or death. Here's where the concept of *vigilance* comes screeching to the fore-front. Like pain, vigilance is an evolutionary function designed to protect us from harm. Once a potential threat is perceived, the nervous system flips into a hypervigilance mode. Vigilance is believed to be co-governed by several connected areas of the brain, including both the left prefrontal cortex and the *amygdala*, an almond-shaped structure just under the temporal cortex that processes emotions, especially emotions that are important, like danger and euphoria.

The term *vigilance* has varied definitions, but the most common usage includes "sustained attention" or "chronic alertness." Having a brain region that considers potential dangers and causes us to engage in active vigilance likely helped our ancestors pass their genes down the line; they were less likely to be eaten by a lion, for instance, or attacked by a neighboring tribe.

Sexual pleasure has been shown to decrease vigilance; it allows us to kick back and let go. This connection between pleasure and vigilance works both ways though. In order for arousal to build into an orgasmic state, we must feel safe enough to let go and open up to sensation. We can only experience this feeling of safety when the state of vigilance is calm.

On the other hand, when vigilance becomes hyperactive due to either actual or perceived danger, our brains become filled with hormones like *adrenaline* and *cortisol*. These hormones are designed to help us remove ourselves from the distressing situation—but they are also known libido killers.[29]

So, what happens when we're stuck in hyperactive vigilance mode, which can happen after all sorts of things, such as an accident, trauma, a major life change, or stress accumulated over time? Once those neural pathways are ingrained, it's like we're stuck in the jungle with only one way out. Over time, this leads to increased anxiety, depression, and chronic tension, all decreasing our ability to respond to pleasurable sensations. This is, in part, why a little wine may help raise libido, since it also lowers vigilance. But it also shows us why that classic advice, "Just relax and have a glass of wine," misses the point entirely. Just like women with a history of chronic pelvic floor tension actually *can't* "just relax," neither can women "just let go" of the grip of hypervigilance without first feeling both emotionally and physically safe.

Tension during sex, therefore, is a strong impediment in our ability to access sexual pleasure. Susana, Dee's client, likely developed pelvic floor tension in response to her urinary tract infections and the subsequent treatments she received as a child. While it's possible she had tension before the infections started, her body learned to hold more tension over time. In addition, Susana was both physically and emotionally distressed when her urethra was dilated by her pediatrician. There's a pretty good chance this frightening and humiliating experience, though entirely well-meaning, created an association between genital touch and misery.

Dee realized that Susana's care was going to be multifaceted. Releasing tension throughout her body would be a big part of her treatment.

On her first visit, the following prescriptions were given. Today, ...
offer them to anyone who is experiencing any type of pain with sex.

Prescription 2

A New Way to Breathe

We breathe automatically, without thinking about it. You may have
been told to breathe deeply to relax or to alleviate pain, but if you
don't practice it, it won't come naturally. We suggest practicing
this technique regularly—ideally, each morning before getting out
of bed and at night before going to sleep—and returning to this
prescription between future prescriptions as needed.

What You'll Need:

- Three minutes. This exercise is done fully clothed, so
  privacy may or may not be necessary, as long as you can
  concentrate on what you are doing.

- A flat surface.

Let's Get Started!

- Lie down.

- Put your hands on your sides, down low over your ribs. Take
  a deep breath that pushes your ribs out on both sides. You
  should feel your hands move out as your ribs expand. You
  might also feel your lower back push down toward whatever
  surface is beneath you. This may be a familiar to you if you've
  ever been taught how to do diaphragmatic breathing.

- Only your ribs should move; your chest or belly should
  not move upward. *This is not a yoga-style deep belly breath.*
  The goal is to use your ribs and diaphragm to draw air in.

- Now breathe in more and more air, pulling it deep into your lower ribs. You should feel more relaxed as your heart begins to beat more slowly. As you do the breathing, visualize your air going all the way down to the opening of your vagina.

- Once you are comfortable here, breathe in deeply and hold it to the count of five. Then exhale, breathing all the air out. Repeat at least five times.

After you get the process down, use the breathing pattern anytime you feel stress or tension anywhere in your body. It can really make a difference.

Prescription 3

Two Simple Stretches

If you have pain with sex, we suggest practicing these stretches regularly—ideally, each morning before getting out of bed and at night before going to sleep.

What You'll Need:

- Five minutes. These exercises are done fully clothed, so privacy may or may not be necessary, as long as you can concentrate on what you are doing.

- A flat surface.

HIP STRETCHES

Let's Get Started!

The hip muscles lie in close proximity to the pelvic floor muscles.

Dee Hartmann and Elizabeth Wood

Tightness in these muscles can cause and/or be caused by increased tension throughout the pelvis.

1. Lie on your back and pull your right knee across your belly and up toward your left shoulder with both hands. Hold it there for a count of twenty. Don't bounce; just hold. Next, pull your right knee up toward the right shoulder and hold it for twenty counts. Then pull your right knee up and out to the side toward your right arm pit. Hold as before.

2. Repeat the three stretch positions with your left knee— going to your right shoulder, left shoulder, and left armpit—holding each for a count of twenty.

3. Alternate the reps above with each knee, repeating three times with each side.

LOWER BELLY STRETCH

The lower belly stretch is an easy stretch that can release tension in the pelvis. If you have an IUD, please do this gently, putting your fingertips just below the belly button.

Let's Get Started!

• Lie on your back and put your hands on your lower belly. Place both thumbs just above your belly button with your hands flat on your stomach. Let your index fingers come together and touch while the others rest in place just above the bone (pubic bone). Think of making a heart with your thumbs and index fingers on your belly.

• Now, using all your fingertips, scoop down and in (toward your back) and then, with your fingers still deep, lift up on your belly (toward your head). Think of trying to get under your belly button to lift it up and out. Be gentle—this should not cause any discomfort!

- As you lift and stretch, you are releasing tension on a series of ligaments that support the urethra, bladder, and pelvic floor muscles, encouraging them to relax.

- Scoop and hold for a count of ten. Repeat three times.

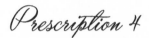
Prescription 4

Two Ways to Mobilize Your Pelvic Floor

These two active exercises will further release tension in the pelvic floor muscles. If you have pain with sex, we suggest practicing them regularly—ideally, each morning before getting out of bed and at night before going to sleep.

What You'll Need:

- Five minutes. These exercises are done fully clothed, so privacy may or may not be necessary, as long as you can concentrate on what you are doing.

- A flat surface.

BRIDGING

Lifting into a bridge tightens muscles on your backside. Coming back down relaxes those muscles, which encourages the muscles inside the pelvis to do the same.

Let's Get Started!

- Lie on your back on a firm surface, such as a couch, a yoga mat, or directly on the floor. Do not do this exercise on a bed or with a pillow under your head.

- Bend both knees up and put your feet flat on the floor. Keep your feet in line with your hips—no wider, no narrower—and directly below your knees.

- Squeeze your buttocks and slowly lift your hips up toward the ceiling until your body is up high enough that your knees, hips, and shoulders are in a straight line.

- Hold for a count of ten. Repeat three times.

PELVIC FLOOR MUSCLE EXERCISES

You have probably heard of pelvic floor muscle exercises, often referred to as "Kegel exercises." Learning to control the muscles as they contract and relax is important—in fact, the letting go is the most important part of the exercise.

Let's Get Started!

- Squeeze and hold on the inside, from the front of your pelvis all the way to the back, like you are trying to hold back pee and gas.

- Then, let go completely. You should be able to feel both the squeeze up and in as well as the letting go, which is down and out. Do this several times to know what it feels like. Letting go of tight muscles isn't always easy, especially if they've been overly tight for a long time. By actively squeezing your muscles, you encourage the nervous system to better release them. Letting go all the way is the end goal!

- Once you can feel the squeeze and letting go, squeeze in and hold to the count of five before letting go.

- Next, tighten the muscles in a series of five small squeezes. You may have heard this called "elevator Kegels." Start with a little squeeze and then, without letting go, squeeze a little bit more, then a little bit more, a bit more, and one last little squeeze. By the last squeeze, all the muscles should be contracting as much as they can. Once you get here, let go all the way. Feel the pelvic floor muscles relax.

- Repeat the previous two steps, alternating the squeeze and hold with the five quick squeezes. Try this several times, feeling the muscles inside begin to relax more each time you let go.

- Repeat this routine daily. Eventually, try to work up to doing the pelvic floor muscle exercise routine for ten minutes a day, splitting it between five minutes in the morning and five minutes at night.

- If you are having trouble doing this or it is causing more pain, go back and repeat the other prescriptions in this chapter before trying again. The pelvic floor exercises should not, we repeat, SHOULD NOT increase pain or tension.

Prescription 5

Use a Vibrator for Muscle Tension Release

Active vibration is often used therapeutically. Remember, many vibrating sex toys are coyly marketed as "massagers," and there's a reason for that: even in the areas that aren't associated with sexuality, vibration can be a pleasant way to release muscle tension. As with calming tension anywhere, a vibrator can help decrease tension in the pelvic floor muscles. Doing so can interrupt your brain's sensory perception of pain, teaching you to feel the vibration instead of the pain. So, in this case, we recommend using a tool that vibrates—

either a sex toy or massager—around your vulva. It's important to note that while this may feel *really* good, we encourage you to not move the vibrator to the area inside your labia at this time, but rather to keep it moving around on the outside. The goal is to have pleasurable sensations throughout your entire vulva.

What You'll Need:

- Five minutes of complete privacy. While this is technically not a self-pleasuring practice, it may well look like one.

- A vibrating massager, usually found online or at a sex toy shop. While we love good vibrators, really any vibrator in any shape will do; in this capacity, it will be used to simply relax the muscles, not for sexual stimulation.

- Lube. We suggest natural oils if you'd like—coconut, olive, or almond oil. Water- or silicon-based lube works well too. Be sure to check the manufacturer's recommendations to find lubes that are compatible with their vibrators.

Let's Get Started!

- Apply lube to the vibrator.

- Lie flat on your back with your knees pointed up or resting out to the sides. Use pillows under your knees if that's more comfortable.

- Hold the vibrator firmly to your pubic bone, which is the easily accessible bone just underneath your mons pubis, and switch it on. Notice how far down into your vulva or down your legs you can feel the sensations of the vibration.

- Begin to move the vibrator slowly around the mons and then around the vulva without going inside to the vagina or over the clitoris. Pause anywhere that you feel tension and see if you can get it to let go.

- Do this for five minutes or more.

Repeat this for several days in a row and notice how the tension has changed. Continue to do this as many times as you like.

Moving out of Pain and into Pleasure

Throughout this chapter, we explored the relationship between pain and pleasure. We looked at how the medical world identifies sexual pain, how pain works in the brain, and introduced many of the common causes. We also looked at how tension works in both the mind and the body, and how unconsciously holding tension in either or both areas can affect our ability to feel pleasure. You may have been a bit unsure at the start, much like Susana whom you met at the beginning of this chapter. She was skeptical whether the simple exercises Dee prescribed could really help. But she soon found that, simple as they are, they are highly effective. We hope you agree.

As you begin to explore how pleasure and pain work together, you'll start to awaken your own sensuality. The two go hand in hand. In the next chapter, we'll look at sensuality all on its own, leaving sexuality aside for the time being. We'll discuss how, as women, we are socialized to disconnect from our senses and how we can restore that connection to experience the deepest sensual pleasure throughout our lives.

CHAPTER THREE

Awakening Your Sensuality

A Note from Elizabeth:

Laura came to me on the recommendation of a friend. She had recently attended an all-women's gathering where a lot of the conversation focused on the great sex the other women were having. Laura was shocked to hear her friends talking about having the best sex of their lives in their fifties. They talked about having multiple orgasms, joked about their headboards banging against the walls, and discussed the latest advancements in USB-chargeable vibrators. Laura found herself gripping her wine glass tighter and tighter, unable to relate. One friend had sensed Laura's discomfort and asked her to meet for coffee the next day. By the bottom of their first cup, Laura had my card in hand.

"I just never really got it, I guess," Laura told me. "I love my husband, and I'm glad we had our kids, so obviously sex is a good thing...but I don't understand what all the hype is about. After hearing my friends, though..." She laughed. "I want what they're having!"

I asked Laura about her early sexual experiences. While there was romance, the experiences weren't particularly tit-illating for Laura. She and her husband loved each and had sex regularly. He was able to bring her to orgasm, but there were no "fireworks"; rather, her orgasms were sort of ho-hum and brought more relief than actual pleasure. Though she enjoyed feeling intimate with him, the disparity between his pleasure and her own was palpable, and she often felt lonely afterward. "I'm having good sex, and I can come, so what am I complaining about?" she asked. When he traveled on business, Laura often used her ancient vibrator to quickly reach orgasm. Even with that, she said, "The fireworks are still missing, but having an orgasm helps me fall asleep."

Laura noted that she wasn't a "touchy-feely" person, and though she was raised in a loving household, her parents had avoided expressing their emotions and rarely touched each other, or her, in a show of affection. Her mother told her sex is for making babies and that men enjoyed it while women, more or less, had to tolerate it.

Laura described herself as socially active; she chaired events for the school association, did some fundraising, and was in a bridge club. I was happy to hear that Laura enjoyed her life but noticed that none of these hobbies involved much movement. Laura said she really didn't like exercising, yoga, or dancing. She told me she wasn't all that comfortable in her body and really didn't enjoy others' touch. As she spoke, her voice was devoid of excitement and her facial expression didn't change.

While it's always hard to determine the root of someone's problem in a single conversation, I began to develop a hunch that Laura was shut off from all of her senses. While she reported a moderate amount of physical satisfaction with sex, she never described a sensual connection to it. In short, I felt that Laura had lost touch with her sensuality. It was natural that her sexuality was suffering as a result. As I asked her questions, Laura, too, noted that she was rarely tapped into her five senses—not only during sex but also throughout her days. A certain spark was missing from her life, and she wanted to know if she could find it.

Over the years, we have seen countless women who have trouble connecting to their sensuality. It keeps them from enjoying a wide variety of nonsexual pleasures and affects their sexuality as well. Sensuality is one way to experience pleasure. In our opinion, it's the best way because it requires us to shift our attention inward to focus on the experience of the five senses. When we actively engage with our senses, we come to realize that pleasure is available to us in every moment. But without sensuality, pleasure—sexual and otherwise—is often limited. When we don't experience the full range of our senses, we become disconnected from our sensuality, and pleasure becomes more a set of thoughts than a set of experiences.

This chapter will explain what we mean by "disconnected." It will delve into what sensuality is, how it differs from sexuality, and how it relates to pleasure. Then it will teach you how to reengage your own sensuality by coming back to your senses and restoring the pleasure in your body. It's about relishing in your senses—and by that, we mean all five of them: sight, sound, smell, taste, and touch. Eventually, this will affect how you experience your sexuality, but in this chapter, we are focusing solely on finding nonsexual sensual pleasure.

We'll start by defining how we use the words *sensual* and *sensuality*. *Sensual* means something that is pleasing to the senses. *Sensuality* is the pleasurable pursuit and enjoyment of the senses. We experience sensuality for the sake of pleasure. Sensual pleasure happens when we feel positive sensations happening in our bodies, which occurs naturally when we're doing something we enjoy. That's what feeling good is all about!

At the heart of sensuality are the five senses. Humans get a tremendous amount of information through *sight*, our most dominant sense. Our eyes perceive rays of light, which the brain translates into colors, shapes, and more. The sense of *sound* comes through the inner ear, which detects vibration that the brain converts into pitch, tone, and volume. Our sense of *smell* is closely linked with memory and emotion and helps us appreciate the flavor of food. Our mouths have the ability e five basic *tastes*—salty, sweet, sour, bitter, and umami. And we have the sense of *touch*, which is perceived primarily through the skin but also through the structures that lie beneath it.

When we take in sensory information, our brains immediately go to work categorizing, defining, and deciphering it. We decide whether it's appealing or not appealing and whether we want more or less of that sensation. When we're in touch with our senses, we generally gravitate toward what we like and away from what does not please us. It's instinctive; we don't have to think about it.

Despite our natural ability to experience things sensually, we often close the door on our senses. As a result, we stop paying attention to the sensations happening in our body. Our senses are always active. Every minute we make choices, whether we attune to them or not, both consciously and unconsciously. If we habitually tune them out, we have a tendency to get stuck in a rut.

So, if your sensuality is stuck on a low setting, we have good news for you: you can turn it up to high. We believe experiencing *all five* senses adds to your sensual well-being in numerous ways. We know this professionally from guiding women like Laura back home to their senses. The results have been, well, *sense*-ational!

As we progress through this chapter, we'll explore how women have disconnected from their senses. Then, we'll look at how this disconnect relates to both physical and emotional pain. Finally, we'll describe the connections between arousal, pleasure, and sensuality. You'll finish this chapter with tools to help you rediscover your sensual pleasure, which is not only the precursor to getting in touch with sexual pleasure; it's also a simple shift in focus that will fundamentally change the way you experience life.

The Disconnect

Children's sensory exploration is natural and helps them navigate the world. In their innocence, they often cross the boundaries of what's safe. "Don't put that in your mouth!" a mother says to her toddler who's holding a penny in her hand. "Don't touch that!" warns a father who sees his child reaching for the hot stove. Innocently, kids make a mess finger painting and playing in the mud and cause lots of noise by banging on pots and pans. They wiggle in their chairs at school, enjoying movement as they resist sitting still. And many children (both boys *and* girls) touch between their legs because it feels good and is soothing, not unlike rubbing their blanket on their noses as they go to sleep. Children are delightfully sensory—unless they are taught not to be.

Parents and childcare providers help young ones learn the difference between acceptable and unacceptable behaviors and how to avoid physical harm—the candle that burns or the fluffy dog who bites. In most cases, corrections are done in the best interest of the child and without ill intent; however, when a child is told they are bad or wrong even when doing something naturally and playfully childlike, the message can be confusing. Something different may land in the child's psyche. To them, corrections—positive or negative—may mean, "I am doing something wrong or bad," which is then perceived as, "I am wrong. I am bad." Boom! There's the disconnect from the innocent and natural enjoyment of our senses.

For many, a disconnect happens early and gets stronger over time. It is often solidified by the time of adolescence. Think of the self-conscious teenager whose father tells her that continuing to eat ice cream will make her fat. Shamed and embarrassed, she decides she'll never eat ice cream again. What about the boy who swears off listening to the radio after his eighth-grade crush tells him he has terrible taste in music? These types of experiences can be damaging and contribute to a conscious disconnect from something that was otherwise pleasurable.

It's important to point out that the disconnect can happen on either end of the spectrum. In other words, we can stuff ourselves with chocolate cake just as easily as we can deny ourselves any and all sweets. We want to be clear that getting in touch with your sensual nature doesn't mean gorging yourself on fried food, dancing until blisters start to form, or—as one of Dee's clients once did—having multiple orgasms till her toes went numb. It's about reaching a healthy balance. Experiencing any one of the five senses doesn't necessarily need to be extreme for us to notice it. To the contrary, if you're in touch with your sensuality, the entire range is available for you to experience: subtle, neutral, and intense. When we're sensually connected, we'll seek out pleasure—but we'll also have appropriate limits, because too much of a good thing can become something not so good. The prescriptions in this chapter aim to teach you that through personal experience. Our hope is that after working with them, you'll order chocolate cake if you want it, enjoy each yummy bite until you're satisfied, and then put the fork down, regardless of what chocolatey gooeyness is still on the plate.

When we've lost interest in doing things that make us feel good, it's often because we have ignored or disconnected from our five senses and the positive messages they provide. When this happens, we don't relish in the sensory delights around us; rather, we go through our days somewhat numb.

A Note from Elizabeth:

Remember in Chapter Two when we talked about vigilance and feeling safe? It's important enough to mention again. When we feel unsafe or uncomfortable, it is hard to feel turned on. I know for myself the safer and more comfortable I feel, the more pleasure I experience.

What I'm talking about is emotional safety. Being there opens us to the possibility of pleasure. As reported by the BBC News, a study conducted in 2003 at the University of Groningen showed that wearing socks improved a woman's ability to achieve orgasm.[30] Uncomfortably cold feet triggered parts of a woman's brain associated with fear and anxiety. "Let them have socks," I say, and make socks the hot new accessory!

Here's the delicious rub: the connection also works another way—the more turned on we are, the safer and more com-

fortable we feel. When we're living a pleasure-filled life, we simply don't sweat the small stuff.

Turning yourself on through sensual pleasure on a regular basis helps tamp down vigilance, leaving you feeling more at home in your body, improving your self-esteem, and helping you be more in tune with the flow of life. Your partner, friends, and maybe even your kids might notice that you're calmer and at more ease.

That's why embodying your senses is so important. It's about having a real mind-body connection to the experiences and sensations you feel. This gives you the ability to weather a wide spectrum of what life throws your way.

How the Disconnect Relates to Sex and Pain

We can also experience disconnects in response to physical pain. This can include sexual pain as well as pain from other things. When there's any type of pain, pleasure takes a back seat and rightly so. It's hard to get excited and aroused when pain is getting you down. (In other words, "Not tonight, dear; I have a headache" is *real*!) Pain becomes the focus of our attention, overwhelming our every thought. We believe that emotional pain can sometimes exacerbate the physical pain many women have with sex. Pain has the capacity to take us totally out of our bodies.

A Note from Dee:

Chronic sexual pain can increase the disconnect. I've seen women who have disregarded their sensuality for a variety of reasons, such as poor body image, anxiety, or depression, causing psychological pain that contributes to this disconnect. What I want to talk about here is how chronic vulvar pain impacts a woman's connection to her sensual self.

When women experience pain at the vulva, the very thought of anything touching it and making the pain worse creates anxiety. Their world becomes smaller and smaller as they avoid anything that might increase their pain. They shy away from being touched sexually, sitting on a bicycle seat, wearing tight clothing, or inserting a tampon. Like anyone with sexual pain, over time, this behavior becomes the accepted "norm."

Women often withdraw from their partners just when they need tender and loving support the most. They distance themselves from any hugging, kissing, or touching in fear of inviting sexual intimacy. Rejecting their partners again and again wreaks havoc on the couple's intimacy. Women find themselves avoiding sexy lingerie, making excuses to go to bed early and alone, and withdrawing completely from any type of touch, whether sexual or not.

On the flipside, women without partners often avoid relationships for all the same reasons. Even if they deeply desire to be with someone, they're often too frightened to make themselves available. "Who wants to date somebody who can't have sex?" was something I heard over and over again in my clinic. Pain with sex doesn't just keep women from having sex; it keeps many from dating at all.

Women worry they'll never get pregnant because they can't have sex. If they make the decision to try to conceive, their anxiety over the pain it will cause is overwhelming. Many who have been able to have a child and want another, can't bear the thought of their vulvar pain possibly worsening after the baby is born. Many women stop exercising because sweating is irritating to their tissues, stop swimming because the chemicals in the water burn their vulva, or stop walking briskly because the friction hurts too much. One woman I treated quit her job and became a recluse because her vulvar pain was so severe.

I realized that many women avoid celebrating much of what it means to be a woman. Many of them used to be dancers, athletes, and enthusiastic lovers, while others only dreamed of the opportunity to be active and make love. One of the most heartbreaking emotions these women express is their anguish over the fear of forever being alone. Fact is, women with vulvar pain don't just lose out on sex; they lose out on so much of life. Disconnecting from their bodies is a reasonable response to being trapped by pain in a place they'd rather not be. Unfortunately, there's often a trade-off that comes with that disconnect: food tastes bland, music sounds monotone, and touch feels like sandpaper on their skin. In the end, women lose the desire and ability to feel pleasure.

If you've used any of these coping strategies, I totally understand. We're here to help you become all you want to be.

When pain is chronic, attempting to avoid any and all sensations can feel like a perfectly good solution. If you are in chronic pain and experiencing a disconnect between you and the sensations in your body, please know this is a common strategy. Our goal is to help you create pleasurable sensations throughout your body. Like a muscle that has grown weak from misuse, we want to help you reconnect to your body through your senses. We refer to that as *embodiment*.

Embodiment is the antidote to disconnect. It requires us to be fully aware of the body, and to be present to how it feels. It's about acknowledging high and low sensations and paying attention to them rather than ignoring them. Without such embodiment, life can be dull and depressing, keeping us from being present to what's happening moment by moment. This is especially true when it comes to sex.

Having sex when we aren't embodied can foster distrust, anxiety, and a sense of loneliness. If our partners are enjoying themselves and we aren't (or, worse, pretending that we are), sex can be alienating and heartbreaking. Instead of bringing us closer, sex without pleasure can create distance between us. And when you compound that with a hypersexualized world where images of mind-blowing sex are used to sell everything from entertainment to health and hygiene, the realization that you're not having mind-blowing sex can be emotionally painful. In order to have greater access to both arousal and pleasure, we need an embodied connection to our sensuality. Such a connection spurs a special kind of alchemy, something we call the *Feel-Good Triad.*

The Feel-Good Triad

Great synergy emerges when arousal, pleasure, and sensuality come together. The three working together form what we call the *Feel-Good Triad.* Discovering your own feel-good triad will help you become more embodied—and yes, eventually it will lead to better sex, though that's only a small part of our aim.

Arousal is a general term, but it is often used to describe sexual arousal. We'll cover that in the next chapter, but here we're talking about arousal as *the physiological and psychological state of being awakened* or *of sense organs being stimulated to a point of perception.* Becoming aroused wakes up any one sense to something that wasn't there before—anything at all, as simple as a friend putting her hand on our shoulder or a good smell wafting from a restaurant window as we walk by. Such stimuli, subtle or intense, put the brain in a state of readiness by sparking changes in the autonomic nervous system and the endocrine system, making our heart rate increase, our breath quicken, and our hormones begin to flow. The goal of arousal is to wake us up and make us wonder, "Hello! What's that new stimulation?" In an attempt to answer the question, our sense organs become more active, receiving more and more input from the stimulus as our awareness increases.

From our perspective, the desired outcome of arousal is pleasure. In other words, it's more pleasing to smell a blooming rose than it is to smell the garbage sitting in the trash can. *Pleasure* is physical and/or emotional enjoyment. It can be experienced either alone or with other people. It's about joy, satisfaction, and personal fulfillment. And it's good for you; it makes you smile! As sex therapist Stella Resnick writes, pleasure is everything from "Aliveness, Activity, Awe" to "Zestful, Zealous, Zippy"![31]

Sensuality is the third leg of the triad. Think of it like the luscious alcohol that infuses the spongy layer of the best tiramisu. Sensuality truly saturates arousal and pleasure, making both richer. Our five senses can help us become aroused and experience pleasure, which opens the doorway to an array of positive experiences that are just not available when we're disconnected.

Because sensuality plays such a key role, it's imperative that we fire up the senses, habitually teaching ourselves to experience them more fully. We have to do this *despite all the forces* that keep us from doing so: our busy schedules; the intrusion of technology; the responsibilities of parenting, work, or both. It's also important to dispel the cultural conditioning that tells us that exploring sensuality is silly and selfish.

Once you embrace your senses, you'll join the ranks of countless women who have embodied their pleasure and whose arousal went through the roof. This shift into their sensuality has had a significant impact on the rest of their lives. These women know, deep in their bones, what they want to say, do, be, and ultimately achieve. And once found, their embodied pleasure is the catalyst that helps them become who they truly want to be. Through the Feel-Good Triad, they successfully found themselves.

By the way, we're not alone in knowing this; there are some amazing teachers out there who call embodied pleasure *turn-on*. Elizabeth notes that tantric and Taoist practitioners have been talking about it for centuries, which she'll tell you more about in Chapter Four. Our take on it is that turn-on is all about developing a deep and ongoing relationship with the Feel-Good Triad.

Do you see the gravity of what we're suggesting here? We hope so, because what we're recommending is actually quite major. We're asking you to shift your personal paradigm. We want you to live fully embodied by intentionally stoking your arousal, pleasure, and sensuality. And eventually, we want living this way to become second nature.

So from this point forward, we're going to teach you how to connect with and embody your senses. We believe it will change your relationship with pain, sex, your partner, and *your whole life*. But lest we get ahead of ourselves, we'll start with a few preliminary prescriptions, listed below.

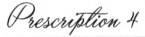

Explore Your Senses

The purpose of this exercise is to help you start identifying what you like and don't like through your five senses. Instead of sitting down in one go and exploring everything at once, try focusing on one sense per day. The goal is to go about your day as normal, integrating the awareness of that sense into everything you do.

What You'll Need:

- A journal and a pen.

Let's Get Started!

- This is a five-day prescription. Use these prompts, one for each day:

   1. Sight: Identify what you like visually. Perhaps you prefer sculpture to painting, bright colors to earth tones, or the sights of the city skyscraper to country

fields awash with spring flowers. How about a star-filled sky at night? Pay attention to what you like for aesthetic reasons alone.

2. Smell: Journey through your spice rack, the perfume counter at the local department store, or the floral section at the grocery store and identify which scents you enjoy. Which ones do you avoid?

3. Taste: Do you enjoy spicy or sour? Sweet or salty? Does your taste change during the day or depending on your mood? Experiment with strong and subtle flavors to determine what you like most.

4. Sound: Do you gravitate toward hip-hop or rap? Country versus classical? Loud or soft noises? Do wind-chimes relax or annoy you? Take notice of the background noises that fill your everyday life.

5. Touch: What fabrics do you like against your skin? How does it feel when you shampoo your hair, dry your body with a towel, or rub lotion into your skin? What speed and pressure do you naturally use to do these daily activities? Pay particular attention to how it feels when you're naked, as bare skin is more sensitive to touch.

• In the morning, take a moment to jot down which of the five senses you'll be working with for that day.

• Then, put heightened awareness on that sense throughout the day. Notice the intricacies of what attracts and repels you. Notice what you naturally gravitate toward. Notice when you like things in an extreme way (maybe it's not just that you like things spicy, you like the burn inside your mouth!) and how what you like changes with circumstances throughout the day. Do you like to play loud music in your car—but reach to turn it down when trying to find a parking spot? Notice how your mood effects what you like. Simply notice. Don't make any judgments.

- At the end of each day, write down what you noticed. What did you learn about that particular sense? What did you learn about yourself? What did you enjoy the most? The least? How did you feel during the exploration? Was it fun? Was it boring? Did any memories come to the surface? Any emotions? Everything is OK; remember, it's an exercise to awaken you to your senses.

- Repeat this five-day process as many times as you like! Practice, practice, practice. It will make a difference, and the more you do it, the more you'll enjoy it.

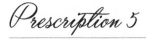

Wake Up Your Pelvis

This sensory practice will increase both your psychological and physiological arousal. Psychologically, it feels good (well, at first it usually feels awkward…but you'll get there!) and brings your awareness to the pelvic region. Physiologically, it increases the blood flow in all the muscles of the pelvic floor, and that is the start of arousal.

What You'll Need:

- Fifteen-plus minutes of complete privacy.

- A stereo and access to some fun music. Play around on a streaming service or create your own playlist that suits your fancy.

- Enough space to move; you don't need a full dance studio, but pushing some furniture back in your living room may be useful.

- Optional: A yoga mat.

Let's Get Started!

- First, repeat the stretches in Prescription 3. These will help you warm up.

- Then, come to all fours with your knees as wide as your hips, your feet directly behind your knees, and your hips at a right angle. Your elbows should be slightly bent so they don't lock. You can spread your fingers out wide with your palms on the floor or, if that hurts your wrists, prop yourself up on your fists with your wrists straight. If getting on your hands and knees is difficult, you can always lean forward against a counter to do the exercise.

- Begin to do the yoga pose known as "cat/cow." As you inhale, allow your belly to relax toward the floor as your shoulders and hips move upward, arching your back. Your pelvic floor muscles relax a bit as you do this. Without straining your neck, look up. Then, as you exhale, lift upward from the center of your spine and tuck your tailbone under as your pelvic floor muscles tighten. Look down and back toward your breasts. You should look like a cat from a Halloween decoration. Continue to move back and forth like this with your breath. It should feel nice and relaxing.

- After a few minutes, get up and start your music. You may also want to lower the lights.

- With your feet hip-distance apart, start moving your hips to the music in a circle, as if you were hula-hooping. Experiment by going in both directions, making your hip movements large and small. Close your eyes if you can keep your balance while doing so; if not, just relax your eyelids so you aren't really focusing on anything in particular. Relax your jaw and let your mouth stay comfortably open. Allow yourself to be totally present to the sensation in your hips, feeling them sway to the music. Try moving your hips in a figure-eight, making sure to go in both directions.

- Let your feet start moving with your hips. Move back and forth across the room, exploring whatever space is available to you.

- After a few minutes, begin to write the letters of the alphabet with your hips. See your tailbone as a pencil pointing toward the floor, and move your hips in the shape of each letter, one by one.

- Now, it gets really fun. Think of the words that you used to describe the wonderful sensual things you found in Prescription 4, and "write" them in the air with your hips.

- Allow yourself to be silly or goofy; if you have any inclination to laugh out loud, please follow it! This is supposed to be fun.

- Let yourself go. Feel the sensations deep in your pelvis every step of the way.

- When you're finished, move back to small circles, paying attention to each movement.

- Then turn the music off and lie back down on the floor to absorb all the great work you just did.

- Stay there for several minutes, just feeling the *aliveness* in your pelvic area. Breathe into this. And promise yourself you'll keep going because *this feeling of aliveness is what you have been waiting for.*

Dee Hartmann and Elizabeth Wood

Starting a Sexual Revolution

In this chapter, we introduced the idea that reconnecting to sensuality is imperative to rediscovering your sexual pleasure—it's the beginning of your own personal sexual revolution. We began by exploring why you may have disconnected from your senses. You then learned about the link between this disconnect and pain—both physical and emotional. We went on to explain the Feel-Good Triad of arousal, pleasure, and sensuality. Finally, we offered you prescriptions to help you embrace your senses again. These prescriptions were extremely helpful to Laura as she slowly moved toward embodied sensuality.

This is the beginning of a journey toward sensual pleasure and embodiment. The lessons from this chapter will continue throughout the book as you naturally disconnect and reconnect to your sensory experience, again and again. It's a worthy endeavor that will change your life.

Once you are fully embodied, sexuality can really begin to flourish. Sexual expression is a natural result of sensual awareness. And it's the topic of the next chapter. We'll start by taking a closer look at how sensuality is an essential precursor to sexuality. Then we'll discuss the topic of self-pleasuring and the importance of making it an integral part of your journey. We'll then talk about orgasm—one of the many potential benefits of a self-pleasure practice. Finally, you'll be guided through pleasure calibration. If the thought of self-pleasuring doesn't float your boat just yet, hang tight. It's our hope that you'll climb aboard and enjoy the sail soon enough.

CHAPTER FOUR

(Re)discovering Sexual Pleasure

A Note from Dee:

Mary was in her sixties. She came to me complaining she'd never had an orgasm. She and her husband had been having sex frequently for over twenty years. Mary shared that she relied on him to bring her pleasure but had never explored it by herself. She'd enjoyed their lovemaking and felt moderate levels of arousal, but when her friends told her that sex after menopause was fantastic, she thought for sure she was missing out on something. She came to me because she simply wanted to experience orgasm at least once before she died!

She told me that as her husband aged, he began having difficulty with erections, which was easily addressed with medication. Prior to that, she explained that they always had sex for an "average" amount of time. When I asked her what "average" meant, she told me that, when he was younger, her husband would typically penetrate her for twenty minutes or longer hoping that if he stayed there long enough, she would eventually have an orgasm. Neither one of them understood why this never worked. Since he had been taking the "little blue pill" (Viagra), the time he stayed erect inside her had increased to forty minutes or longer, and still: nothing.

Inside, I was grimacing. Twenty or forty minutes of active thrusting is not "average"; this is a myth perpetuated by porn and misinformed overachievers. I asked her if she liked being penetrated that long and if it was pleasurable. She said the only pain she experienced was from friction. Fortunately, she'd discovered the benefits of lube that made their extended periods of lovemaking tolerable but certainly not more pleasurable.

I asked Mary how she thought I could help. She explained that her doctor had told her she had anorgasmia, *a sexual dysfunction defined by the inability to reach orgasm, and that it required treatment. Her doctor told her there were new medications on the market to address women's problems with sex. Because she wanted a more natural solution, her doctor referred her to me. She really wanted to find a more natural solution.*

After our discussion, I began my physical exam. Mary's pelvic floor muscles felt a little weak, which was typical for a woman her age, and she seemed disconnected from her sensuality. It was clear she would benefit from the pelvic floor muscle exercises we presented earlier in this book, as well as exploring her sensual side. I also made sure to cover most of what she needed to know about her anatomy during the physical exam. I was confident that I could help Mary experience more pleasure in her body and possibly reach orgasm. The plan was to have Mary start by calibrating her pleasure.

L ike Mary, we wanted to make sure that you have all the basics before getting to this point. First, we taught you about your body's design and function and helped you be comfortable while looking at your vulva in the mirror. Next, we gave our best explanation of how pain and tension work in both the body and the brain, and helped you start stretching and exercising the muscles that can cause pain during sex. Then, we explored the treasures of sensuality, which we honestly hope is changing the way you experience being in your body.

Now we believe you are ready to bring all three of those elements together to start exploring sexual pleasure.

This chapter is about awakening—either from a long sleep, or for the very first time—the sexual pleasure that your body was designed to feel. As we see it, you have the right to feel this pleasure. It's uniquely yours. It's a precious gift that we want to help you nurture and cultivate.

As you learned in the last chapter, pleasure is not necessarily sexual—but it can be. According to the Global Advisory Board on Sexual Health and Wellbeing, "Sexual pleasure is the physical and/or psychological satisfaction and enjoyment derived from solitary or shared erotic experiences, including thoughts, dreams and autoeroticism."[32] We often think of sexual pleasure as something that is shared with a partner. Indeed, it can be. If you choose to go that route, Part III of this book is devoted to that aim. But as women, we're often overly focused on the part of our sexuality that is shared with partners—in most of our clients' cases, men—rather than our own.

In truth, there is nothing wrong with solo sexual experiences. Self-pleasuring is great and we highly endorse it. As a matter of fact, we believe the best way to experience and deepen sexual pleasure is, in fact, on your own. Chances are, if you don't know what to do to make yourself feel good, it's pretty tough to teach someone else how to bring you pleasure. Like Dee's grandma used to say, "How can you teach somebody to make the best pineapple upside-down cake if you don't know how to make one yourself?"

Let's face it, it's much easier to figure out what feels good when nobody else is in the room. This eliminates the pressure of having to please someone else.

But before we ask you to explore the self-pleasure prescription, we need to look at a few other important things. We'll start by expanding the continuum of sensuality that we intentionally skipped over in the last chapter: sexual sensuality. Then we'll discuss a silent killer of sexual expression: sexual shame. Finally, we'll discuss the complexity of orgasm. This chapter is juicy and exciting and may make you a little nervous. Keep reading; we're with you!

The Overlap between Sensuality and Sexuality

In the last chapter, we mentioned that sensuality can be sexual. The terms *sensuality* and *sexuality* are often mistakenly used interchangeably, even though the two are distinct phenomena. *Sexuality* has to do with sexual matters including sexual arousal, a person's sexual orientation or preference, and, of course, sexual activity, whether it be for recreation (fun!) or procreation (babies!). A person can be sensual without being sexual. So, too, can a person be sexual without being sensual. We don't encourage the latter, though, because sex is so much better when the senses are invited in to play and are intentionally incorporated in a sexual experience.

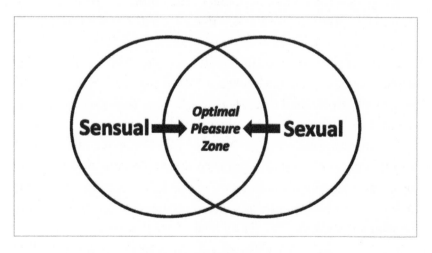

Activating optimal pleasure

The overlap between the two circles above is where sex becomes more fulfilling both physically and emotionally. We can absolutely have sex that feels good (sensual pleasure) without experiencing climax, also known as *orgasm* (sexual pleasure), just like Mary. However, when we engage all of our senses in a sexual experience, we open ourselves up to mind-blowing pleasure. This is precisely why we focused on expanding your sensual experiences in the last chapter. In doing so, it's our hope that being sensual becomes second nature to you, something you don't think about…it just happens. As a result, your sensuality will naturally be involved in your sex play because you will experience just how much better sex feels when your senses are awake and on board. We are committed to helping women everywhere increase the middle section of the Venn diagram where the two circles intersect.

So how do we increase the space within the center segment of the diagram, where sensuality and sexuality overlap? You now know arousal sparks when any one of the five senses is activated. Pleasure is the enjoyable experience of not just sensual arousal but can also be the enjoyable experience of sexual arousal. In Chapter One, we described what happens to the clitoris when it's aroused. And in Chapter Two, we learned that adequate arousal is necessary for penetration to feel good. So let's take it a step further and consider the *type* of arousal that makes sex feel its best: arousal that is pleasing to one or more senses. Put simply, sex is best when the senses are stimulated in a pleasurable way. This pleasure brings arousal, and the more aroused we are, the better the sex.

Connecting sensuality to sexuality, therefore, is a phenomenal way to ignite—or reignite—our own sexual pleasure. An important piece we want you to understand is that by cultivating and feeling how your body responds to sensual, sexual arousal, and pleasure by yourself, the more you'll be able to share that pleasure with your partner. It *has* to start with you, all on your own—not the other way around. We're asking you to take responsibility for your own pleasure. We want you to know first-hand (pun intended) who you truly are sexually. It's this type of embodiment that fuels empowerment. It's hot and sexy!

Shame and Self-Pleasure

Before we discuss self-pleasuring, we need to talk about sexual shame. We've made reference to shame before and want to speak about it here in greater length. In our careers working with women, and as women ourselves, we know just how damaging sexual shame can be. Regardless of their backgrounds, most of the women we have seen experienced some degree of sexual shame; it's unfortunately that pervasive. We've observed that simply discussing self-pleasuring tends to increase women's experience of shame. Note that we're using *self-pleasure* instead of *masturbation* here. For all intents and purposes, the two terms are synonymous, but we're being careful about our language because the root of the word *masturbation* is actually "*to disturb*,"[33] a linguistic connection that we wholeheartedly reject.

Let us be clear: There is nothing, *nothing,* that is inherently wrong, harmful, or disgraceful about self-pleasuring—for men *or* for women.

Self-pleasuring is natural. Although women have practiced self-stimulation for eons, there are many who have never explored their bodies this way. Self-stimulating can start quite early. As we noted in the last chapter, it is completely normal for toddlers or even babies to touch and play with their genitals. Adults are often uncomfortable when they witness a child touching themselves. Some children are sharply reprimanded or outwardly shamed for such behavior, while others are stopped by physical force. What a child learns from these forms of discipline is that they are wrong or bad for doing something that feels good. This can have a detrimental effect, leaving the child unwilling and unable to self-pleasure due to feeling shame or guilt. As a result, many kids struggle against engaging in a behavior that makes things feel so nice because they've been scolded and told it was wrong. The message translates to it is "not right" or "not proper" to give oneself pleasure. If they continue to do so, despite being told not to, the feelings of shame and guilt compound over time.

This is another way we disconnect from our sensuality and the sensual forms of pleasure that we discussed in the last chapter. There's no way to say this except to say it bluntly: in a world where male sexual pleasure takes priority over female sexual pleasure, the disconnect happens disproportionally more so for girls. That's because many girls, even those who come from otherwise progressive backgrounds, are taught that they are not supposed to experience pleasure or enjoy sex. Like Laura, Elizabeth's client whom you met in Chapter Three, they hold the belief that sex is something men enjoy and women more or less tolerate, so feeling desire for sex becomes shameful. Even though Mary, Dee's patient, wasn't consciously ashamed of her sexuality, Dee had a hunch Mary might uncover some degree of shame as she explored sexual experiences on her own.

That's because this shame coincides with girls suppressing the pleasurable sensations they feel in their bodies. It puts them into a loop; by disconnecting from their sensual pleasure, they begin to feel it less, which was precisely what Mary was experiencing. The pleasurable sensations are quashed and ignored in the hope they will just go away. Many girls either stop self-pleasuring or never start. Others feel ashamed but are unable to stop self-pleasuring, so they do it in secret, often resulting in negative thoughts about their "naughty" behavior.

So what happens when we harbor such shame? Pleasure becomes something to avoid. If we do experience it, it can cause emotional distress. Later in life, it may make it harder to reach orgasm because we never explored how to make it happen. We then rely on our partner(s) to figure it out and "bring us" the pleasure we desire—a job that, frankly, *is not theirs*. As women, we need to take responsibility for our own pleasure. We can't wait for the perfect partner to show up and rock our world—or our clitoris—without any input on our part. It's up to each one of us to figure out how our body works. Then, if we want to involve a partner, all we need to do is to bring them up to speed.

This is why our next step is to guide you through experiencing sexual pleasure on your own. This is a profound act of love and self-acceptance. We'll start slow here, really slowly. But we expect huge effects when you follow through. In this moment, you may not know what feels good to you and what doesn't. Perfect. It's a great place to start!

Please know that this chapter's prescription may bring up a host of emotions. You could find that it makes you want to cry either with sorrow or joy. You could find that you need a little more time for yourself to write, walk, create, or otherwise process the feelings that may emerge. All of that is a normal part of the process, and a part that many women experience as they start experimenting with solo sex. Remember, our hope is that you open more and more to sexual pleasure.

But not everyone will have an emotional experience. No matter what you feel after completing the prescription at the end of this chapter, don't be surprised if you want to do it again…and again… and again.

On Orgasm

Remember Mary, whom you met at the beginning of the chapter? She was having enjoyable sex with a husband she loved; however, what she wanted was to have an orgasm. But what exactly is an orgasm? Like many women, Mary had no idea.

Here's where we take a stab at the elusive and constantly evolving definition of *orgasm*. Most people define it as a peak of sexual excitement followed by a release of tension that was built up during arousal and stimulation. It is a discharge of accumulated energy at the height or climax of the sensation. Practitioners from various disciplines use different factors when defining *orgasm*. For instance, most medical practitioners use physiological changes in the body as an underlying foundation for a definition, while psychologists and those in the field of mental health use emotional and cognitive changes. But overall, there is no consensus on exactly where the female orgasm starts—let alone what it actually *is*.

As our sexual health mentor, Dr. Domeena Renshaw, said, "Orgasm is a whole-body experience; it happens in both the mind and the body!"[34] The science suggests that this is true; both the psychologists and the medical doctors are right, and fortunately, we now have science to back this up. Unfortunately, the news has been slow to reach the general public.

The bottom line is that we can't give you *one* definition of *orgasm*. Think of an orgasm the way you might think of a snowflake. While a snowflake is a snowflake, each one has a beautifully different pattern created in response to a whole host of conditions.

How a woman defines her orgasm is layered with rich complexity and is determined by what she actually thinks an orgasm is. Seriously, it's true. As one paper states,

> The distinction between different orgasms, then, is not between sensations of the external clitoris and internal vagina, but between levels of what a woman understands a 'whole' orgasm to consist of. This depends on the experience with direct stimulation of the external clitoris, internal clitoris, and/or cervix, but also with knowledge of the arousing and erotic cues that predict orgasm, knowledge of her own pattern of movements that lead to it, and experience with stimulation of multiple external and internal genital and extra-genital sites (e.g. lips, nipples, ears, neck, fingers, and toes) that can be associated with it.[35]

Women's orgasms, the research shows us, vary widely not only from woman to woman, but in how and where they're happening within the same woman not only as she ages, but they also differ depending on whom she's partnered with. The paper goes on:

Orgasms do not have to come from one site, nor from all sites; and they do not have to be the same for every woman, nor for every sexual experience even in the same woman, to be *whole* and *valid*. And it is likely that such knowledge changes across the lifespan, as women experience different kinds of orgasms from different types of sensations in different contexts and/or with different partners. Thus, what constitutes a 'whole' orgasm depends on how a woman sums the parts and the individual manner in which she scales them along flexible dimensions of arousal, desire, and pleasure. The erotic body map a woman possesses is not etched in stone, but rather is an ongoing process of experience, discovery, and construction which depends on her brain's ability to create optimality between the habits of what she expects and an openness to new experiences. Most importantly, the application of a restricted reproductive model of male ejaculation to understanding the cause and effect of women's orgasms only serves to obfuscate and hide the truly remarkable variety of orgasmic experiences a woman can have.[36]

Not even the experts could agree on an all-encompassing single definition of the female orgasm. After a comprehensive review of the literature that's out there on the human female orgasm, the authors of another well-documented article state that "most of those defining orgasm use reported or observed physical changes (usually muscular and cardiovascular), with an emphasis that this is the culmination or most intense moment of sexual arousal."[37] This is why we often use the words *orgasm* and *climax* interchangeably. The authors of that study went on to further define the female orgasm as follows:

...a variable, transient peak sensation of intense pleasure, creating an altered state of consciousness, usually with an initiation accompanied by involuntary, rhythmic contractions of the pelvic striated circumvaginal musculature, often with concomitant uterine and anal contractions, and myotonia that resolves the sexually induced vasocongestion (sometimes only partially) and myotonia, generally with an induction of well-being and contentment.[38]

It appears the one thing all the science agrees upon is that the female orgasm is complex—and deeply personal.

A Note from Dee:

Though I'm not a researcher, I have discussed orgasm with literally hundreds of women, so I'd like to offer my two cents here. The age-old question of how female orgasm happens frequently centers more on "where" they happen rather than "why" or "how" they happen. As you just learned, it is incredibly difficult to declare one specific, universal definition of what climax is.

That said, I can describe the physical changes that happen in the body during sexual arousal and at the time of climax. Your blood pressure, heart, and respiratory (breathing) rates all rise. As arousal builds, blood flow increases within the walls of the vagina, producing and releasing natural lubricant. As you continue to experience a pleasurable build-up of arousal, the toes might begin to curl, muscle tension will increase, and your nipples may become erect. The uterus reacts to heightened states of excitement by lifting up and in, increasing the length of the vaginal canal in preparation for penetration. A whole dose of "feel good" hormones are released, increasing measurable levels of dopamine, serotonin, oxytocin, and endorphins, all pushing you toward what some experience as an altered state of consciousness. It's almost as if at the point of climax, nothing else exists; you are simply floating in space and time.

At the peak of excitement, the pelvic floor involuntarily and rhythmically contracts. Following those contractions, which can last anywhere from thirteen to fifty-one seconds,[39] there's a sense of relaxation and contentment throughout the body. As the pelvic floor muscles relax, so too does the opening of the vagina—it begins to enlarge. Because of this natural phenomenon, I strongly suggest that my pain patients have an orgasm before attempting any type of vaginal penetration. It is in this state that the opening is most malleable and hospitable to being penetrated by a toy, finger, or penis. (And besides, after an orgasm, everything feels better!)

I have a quick story to share about one of my former pain patients who had no idea that healthy pelvic floor function had anything to do with orgasm. Remember that if your pelvic floor muscles don't have the ability to fully contract and relax, the experience of climax is at best compromised and more often than not, impossible. This client spent a month working on pelvic floor muscle exercises that I'd assigned. About four and a half weeks later, she happily reported, "Dee, the exercises really helped! I had an orgasm that went from my waist all the way down to my knees!"

There's also a lot that's happening neurologically during arousal and orgasm. Some areas of the brain are calmed while others become more activated. A bevy of researchers have well documented the changes in brain activity and blood flow across different brain regions. While we can't cover this in detail here, if you are interested, you will find plenty of information (including in-depth analyses of a host of brain scans) online.

Even with all that's written above, there's still a lot that science doesn't know about women's climax. Funding for studies on healthy sexual function and pleasure in women is hard to obtain; research dollars tend to go toward female sexual dysfunction, which might be more profitable to "fix." Elizabeth and I are hopeful that more study on this subject will happen as our culture begins to place higher value on understanding female sexuality.

If you've never had an orgasm, know that you are not alone. Many women, like Mary, report that despite enjoyable sex, they have still not had this experience. And if you can have orgasms, but they feel, well, anti-climactic, you're not alone either. In fact, you may notice that the women we profiled in the first part of this book had trouble with orgasm—some, like Mary, couldn't reach it, while others, like Laura, were still waiting for the fireworks to happen. We've focused on difficulties with orgasm because it's one of the most common complaints women have when they first walk into our offices.

Many women find that they can reach orgasm from one type of stimulation but not another. While scientists are still trying to figure out exactly what types of stimulation are necessary for climax to occur, countless women find that stimulating the clitoris is the most important part of the process. The truth of the matter is that most women do not climax from vaginal penetration alone.[40]

Many women self-stimulate their clitoris with their own hands or a toy during penetration. Some women's partners help with this. Others find that certain positions are more likely to stimulate their clitoris than others, and that these positions help them orgasm while being penetrated. In any case, while many areas can be stimulated to produce orgasm, the only orgasm that matters to you is the one that you make happen. There is no right or wrong way to have an orgasm, and whatever your experience with it may or may not be, you aren't broken, and you don't need to be fixed.

There is another definition for *orgasm* that goes beyond climax and the medical community's understanding, delving into ancient forms of sacred, spiritual sexuality. Elizabeth will explain more:

A Note from Elizabeth:

As Dr. Kenneth Ray Stubbs says, "If we wish to understand orgasm, we must know energy." I agree, and I often cause confusion when I talk about orgasms, because I understand it as something broader than climax; I understand orgasm as a peak release of orgasmic energy.

To better help you understand orgasmic energy, it may help to take you back in time to Taoism and tantra, both sacred traditions based in Eastern cultures. At the heart of these complex philosophies lies an understanding of orgasm that is actually quite simple. Essentially, the ancient masters were working with what is known as orgasmic energy, which is the energetic basis for the concept of turn-on that we presented in the last chapter. It's that creative, unstoppable force that makes us magnetic, fully embodying our pleasure.

According to these traditions, orgasmic energy exists within each one of us, and despite current widespread belief, is not centered in the genital area. Orgasmic energy can be felt throughout the body. If we attune to it, we can feel the energy flowing. This takes practice. Such awareness of what's happening inside the body is called interoception, *the direct communication between the senses and the brain. You feel hungry when there's nothing in your belly, not just because your brain knows it's lunchtime. When you're anxious or nervous and are feeling butterflies in your stomach, that's interoception too. Conscious perception is key; it means we must pay attention to the sensations and acknowledge that they are present within.*

Back to the idea that not all orgasms happen in the genitals: one of the dictionary definitions of orgasm *is "intense excitement."[41] Have you ever experienced a laugh-gasm or even a food-gasm? I have; though I didn't have a genital climax, I found myself so involved in my sensory pleasure that my body released tension, sending waves of energy that I felt from my head to my toes.*

I believe orgasmic energy is one the world's first nutrients. I refer to it as the original superfood. Much like a superfood, orgasmic energy confers health benefits, with few properties considered to be negative. It is an energy that wakes up our creativity, self-confidence, and spontaneity. Orgasmic energy has been described as our life-force and creative energy. As Deepak Chopra has said, "Sexual energy is the primal and creative energy of the universe. All things that are alive come from sexual energy." I agree. Our very existence is dependent on orgasmic energy. Creating life is the most potent outcome of orgasmic energy.

Feeling orgasmic energy doesn't mean that you're sexually aroused all the time; it means you have access to the creative, inspiring energy of orgasm at will. Through activating orgasmic energy—living on a steady diet of the superfood that is orgasm—your whole life can change. This is turn-on. And it can happen regardless of whether it leads to climax. I hope that by broadening your definition of orgasm, you can find orgasm itself—the energy, and the climax—more accessible. And I hope it changes your life, as it has changed mine.

As you begin to engage yourself sexually, we stress that climax should never be considered the only goal. It's about enjoying the entire ride and activating the orgasmic energy Elizabeth introduced above. We want you to live in a space where this energy is so available that climax is just the icing on the cake! Changing the focus from goal-oriented to pleasure-oriented can help to reduce any sense of performance anxiety or desire to "reach" some particular place. It's about the journey, not the destination. This can make the whole experience more pleasurable as you relax and enjoy the sex you're having.

That said, if you want to reach climax (again and again and again), we want to help you.

We'll do that with a self-pleasure practice. We'll start by focusing on something we often use with our clients and patients: *pleasure calibration*. Pleasure calibration was created to measure the changing temperature of your arousal. It's a skill-building tool that allows you to understand and explore the full capacity of your pleasure. Reaching orgasm requires a buildup of turn-on;

it requires your arousal to increase, but not necessarily in a linear fashion. Arousal ebbs and flows, starts and stalls, often remaining still for moments. Remember, climax happens at the peak of sexual excitement. Learning what these different levels feel like in your body and being able to calibrate them goes a long way toward deepening your capacity to experience your entire arousal range. Think of using pleasure calibration like a thermometer measuring degrees from neutral to red hot!

As you try the prescription on the next page, pay attention to how your arousal changes in response to touch using various pressures, locations, and rhythms. Remember, pleasure is a process. It's not like slogging up a hill; it's more like music. Just as the notes of a song go up and down, your pleasure can rise and fall as your orgasmic energy builds.

As you gain experience with this practice, you'll also build and strengthen your neural pathways toward positive sexual experiences. That means if sex has historically been emotionally or physically painful for you, self-pleasuring may help you open new possibilities for sex to feel good.

For this, we've created a six-stage Pleasure Calibration Scale™ to help you track your pleasure along the way:

The Pleasure Calibration Scale™

0 – Ain't nothin' going on here.

1 – Huh. This might be interesting!

2 – Oh! I think I feel something!

3 – Wow! Alrighty then. Let's keep this going!

4 – I'm cooking now! This is amazing!

5 – OMG! Don't stop, don't stop!

And eventually...

6 – Wheeeee! Here I come!

The Pleasure Calibration Scale™

As you engage in your pleasure calibration, notice where you find yourself on the scale, and how easily you are able to move up and down through the stages.

We also encourage you to add in factors that stimulate the other senses, in addition to touch. Turn some music on; light a fragrant candle or use some essential oils; take a long, hot bath; or whatever you like that increases the sensual experience. Whatever flips your skirt works for us! *The one thing we ask of you at this stage is that you do not use a vibrator or a dildo.* We are both fans of sex toys and know they can bring women great pleasure, but for now, we want you to experiment with creating pleasure using nothing but your own touch.

Having the foundation of a solid self-pleasure practice is a key to more pleasurable and fulfilling partnered sex. Research shows that women who have a better understanding of their sexual selves (how they think about themselves as a sexual individual) more easily recognize and acknowledge their sexual needs and are more confident in stating what brings them pleasure in partnered sex.[42]

Prescription 6

Pleasure Calibration, Part A: External Self-Pleasure

Without further ado, we present the first self-pleasuring practice. If you're nervous, that's okay. Excitement is okay too. Perhaps this will be your first time touching yourself this way. If so: *Congratulations!* If you're familiar with self-pleasuring, please humor us by trying it our way for a while. In all cases, go as slowly as you need to go. If you feel this is moving way too fast, we suggest leaving your panties on until you become more comfortable.

During this practice (Part A), we ask that you stay focused on your vulva and not penetrate your vagina. One of the goals of this exercise is for you to feel your body's ascent up the Pleasure Calibration Scale.

What You'll Need:

- Thirty minutes of complete privacy.

- Optional: Extra pillows to prop yourself up.

- Optional: A journal and a pen.

Let's Get Started!

- Undress down to your comfort level (panties on or off).

- Make yourself comfortable in a chair or on a bed. If you are on your bed, you may choose to have your legs extended in front of you or to lie down with knees bent up to the ceiling, with your feet on the mattress. Use the extra pillows to support yourself if necessary.

- Begin by simply placing a cupped hand skin-to-skin or on top of your panties so that the palm is resting on your pubic mound with fingers gently resting over your outer labia covering your vulva.

- Place your other hand over your heart and begin a short series of deep belly breaths or the breathing technique we described earlier.

- Stay here for a few moments and notice any sensation that you might feel between your hand and vulva.

- Let your breath return to its normal rhythm.

- Tune in and notice if you feel heat building under the hand that is resting over your vulva. Perhaps you can sense a slight tingling down below.

- While maintaining contact between your cupped hand and vulva, very slowly and slightly begin to increase the pressure of the cupping of your hand and then releasing it, applying whatever amount of pressure suits you. Gently squeeze and let go. Make sure to take time to explore this sensation for a few minutes.

- Next, if you're sitting in a chair, start a rocking motion by gently rolling your pelvis forward and back. If you're lying on your bed, create the rocking motion by gently curling your low back up from the mattress and then releasing it back down. In both positions, allow your pelvis to move freely beneath your relaxed hand.

- Start experimenting. Try applying different amounts of pressure to your vulva with your hand.

- Explore the speed of your rocking motion. Move faster, slow things down, and then speed up again. Stay with this motion until you begin to feel something. Note where the sensation is in your body and where that sensation may travel.

- Next, try moving your fingers in a wave-like motion over your vulva or move your fingers together side-to-side or in a circle around in one direction and then the other. Using all your fingers, try stroking upward from the bottom of your outer labia to your clitoris on top, exploring what sensations and strokes feel good.

- Feel the arousal energy rise and fall in your body. Notice when it does and where it goes. Does it spread to your vagina? Does it move across your belly or down your arms and legs? Can you feel it in your head?

- See how many different strokes and styles you like and identify all the ways that touch can feel good.

- Spend at least thirty minutes enjoying this exercise, with feeling pleasure as your only goal, regardless of whether you come to climax.

- When you feel complete, lay comfortably on the floor or bed and close your eyes. Let all the good work you've done wash over your body.

- You may choose to journal what you felt, what you noticed, focusing on both your physical and your emotional experiences.

We suggest you practice this several times before moving forward. If there's a noticeable improvement, keep up the good work! If you see no improvement, add a dose of patience and keep going. It takes time to carve a new pathway to pleasure! When you're ready, you can move on to Part B.

Prescription 7

Pleasure Calibration, Part B: Self-Pleasuring with Exploratory Penetration

Your next prescription involves taking your panties off and spending more time touching all the parts of your vulva, including the areas around and inside your vagina. Knowing more about what areas like to be touched and how they like to be touched increases your pleasure on the calibration scale. If you reach climax during this practice, congratulations! But it should not be your goal.

One caveat: In this prescription, we want you to hold off on deep thrusting penetration. Be curious, but stay near the vaginal opening. Move slowly, gently, and gradually as you explore with your finger(s) the sensations of having something just inside your vagina. You're doing great!

What You'll Need:

- Thirty minutes of complete privacy.

- Lube. We suggest natural oils if you'd like—coconut, olive, or almond oil. Or, water-based lube works well too.

- Optional: Extra pillows to prop yourself up.

- Optional: A mirror and good lighting.

- Optional: A towel to put underneath you.

- Optional: A journal and a pen.

Let's Get Started!

- Make yourself comfortable in a chair or on your bed. If on your bed, it's your choice to have your legs extended in front of you or to lie down with knees bent, soles of your feet on the mattress. Use the extra pillows to support yourself. If you like, you can place a towel under your naked bottom.

- Begin by simply placing a cupped hand over your vulva so that the palm is resting on your pubic mound with fingers gently resting over your outer labia. Feel the sensation of just touching yourself, skin to skin.

- Place your other hand over your heart and begin a short series of deep belly breaths or the breathing technique described earlier.

- Stay here for a few moments and notice any sensation that you might feel between your hand and vulva.

- Let your breath return to its normal rhythm.

- Apply lubricant to your fingers and vulva, and with your fingers begin to trace your inner and outer labia using soft, gentle strokes.

- Try gently pulling, tugging, and stroking your inner labia.

- Find your clitoris, and stroke all of it: the head, shaft, hood, and the clitoral bulbs.

- Vary the length, position, and speed of your strokes. Try circles in both directions, long strokes from your vaginal opening to your clitoris, or short, quick strokes over the clitoral glans. With your finger(s) over your clitoris, try pulsing or tapping for variety. Move your fingers around slowly using back and forth, side to side, and up and down motions. Decide what part of your hand to use: fingers, fingertips, or even your palm. There's no wrong way to do this!

- You may note that the head of the clitoris is very sensitive and often doesn't like direct stimulation. If this is the case, it may feel better to stimulate the clitoris and clitoral shaft through the hood. With arousal, the entire clitoris will plump up and change form. The clitoral shaft can be felt underneath the hood as if it were a cocktail straw. Experiment by rolling your fingers back and forth over the shaft to expand areas of pleasure.

- Continue your exploration by moving your fingers down and across your labia using swiping motions with different pressure.

- Periodically take breaks to check yourself out in the mirror. This can be a huge turn-on! Notice how your vulva has changed. Look for a change in color, which is caused by increased blood flow to the area. Can you see that it has visibly changed size, becoming plump and swollen?

- Identify what strokes and speed you like and don't like. Do circles in one direction feel better than circles in another? Do you like different levels of pressure at different moments? Notice everything.

- At this point, your arousal level should be high enough to begin gentle penetration. Remember the Pleasure Calibration Scale? Your calibration should be at stage 3 or 4. If it's not, go back and continue to build arousal until you get there. Don't get discouraged if it doesn't happen the first time. This is a practice and takes time.

- If you are delightfully curious to explore and are craving vaginal penetration, place a relaxed fingertip just inside the opening of your vagina. Hold here, take a deep breath, and don't enter farther just yet. If you experience discomfort, continue to breathe and refocus your attention on your pleasure. If that doesn't work, keep practicing the earlier prescriptions until you are ready to move forward.

- Once you are ready, feel around the vaginal opening, tracing the entire circle with a little pressure. Gently move your finger in a bit deeper, then squeeze your pelvic floor muscles and let them go. Notice what it feels like against your finger. The squeezing and letting go is what happens naturally with orgasm.

- From here, sense whether you'd like to insert your finger inside your vagina any further. If so, with a well-lubricated finger, slowly insert it to your comfort. Slowly move it in and out, exploring just inside the opening. Now go back in and move your finger from side to side, gaining access to more and more pleasure. Notice the warmth, the space, and the texture. Relax and enjoy whatever you want to explore.

- Like you did in the first pleasure calibration exercise, feel the orgasmic energy rise and fall in your body. Notice where it is; does it stay only in the area around your vulva? Does it spread to your vagina? Does it move across your belly or down your arms and legs? Can you feel it in your head?

- Spend at least thirty minutes enjoying this exercise, regardless of whether you experience (or even get close to experiencing) climax.

- When you feel complete, lay comfortably on the floor or bed and close your eyes. Let all the good work you've done wash over your body.

- You may choose to journal what you noticed, focusing on both your physical and your emotional experiences.

Taking Your Pleasure into Your Own Hands

If you just tried self-pleasuring for the first time, you may find that you want to repeat it. If so, you have our full permission! Repeat this as much as you want; as you gain more confidence and comfort, you'll find that you can calibrate your own pleasure more easily, knowing where you are on the scale at any given point in time. If the prescription wasn't particularly thrilling, that's okay, too; these things take time. We believe that self-pleasuring is absolutely essential to establishing or reestablishing a relationship with joyful penetrative sex. But take everything at your own pace; there's no pressure to go any faster than you need to go.

As Mary progressed through the prescriptions above, she reported that she found numerous ways to touch herself that felt good. With a smile on her face and a kick in her step, she told Dee she was now reaching a 5 or 6 on the Pleasure Calibration Scale more frequently. Not only did Mary have her first of many orgasms, she felt energized and more creative. Elizabeth would say this is "life powered by orgasm." While not everyone will have this experience, we know that for many, it is possible. Mary found that the possibility increased when she became comfortable with a self-pleasure practice.

We want to acknowledge that, for a lot of you, this chapter was really big. Self-pleasuring can be a hard thing to do for a lot of women. Throughout the chapter, we looked at the connection between sensuality and sexuality and the disconnect between the two. We discussed how feeling shame impacts sex, and how many women experience increased shame with the idea of self-pleasure. And we presented two views on orgasm—the very topic that may have pushed some of you to pick up this book in the first place. We then offered you a guide, the Pleasure Calibration Scale, to help you measure your pleasure on your own. Lastly, you were given step-by-step prescriptions to develop self-pleasure practices that we suggest you continue using for an indefinite period of time.

This chapter concludes Part I of the book. You may want to stick to this portion of the book and the prescriptions within it for a while before moving on to Part II, which presents more advanced ideas and prescriptions. You may also be ready to move on to Part II right away. No two women are the same, and one way that we hope to increase your agency through this book is by absolutely affirming, again and again, that you do what feels right for you.

In any case, we hope that Part I has given you a much stronger understanding of your body, your pain, your sensuality, and your capacity for sexual pleasure. We hope you're thrilled and filled with new information. We hope you are engaging in pleasurable and arousing experiences, embodied and sensually aware. And we hope that orgasmic energy has started to ripple out, bringing you more joy and aliveness throughout your life.

Believe us when we say: this is just a taste of what's to come.

Part Two

The Advanced Solo
Practices

CHAPTER FIVE

Addressing Your External Influencers

A Note from Dee:

Tara came to me with a common concern: she had no desire for sex. Whenever her husband approached her, she turned away, each time citing a different reason—there was laundry to fold, a dog to walk, kids to feed, and by the way, when was the last time he mowed the lawn? "No matter how many excuses I find, I know the problem is mine," Tara explained. She told me she was looking for a quick fix.

I started with questions about her relationship. Tara's responses spilled over to include the rest of her life. She left a lucrative and interesting career because she was taught that a "stay-at-home mom" was the best mom to be. Although she liked being at home with her kids, who were two and four, she missed the intellectual challenge and camaraderie with her peers. Many of her friends did continue to work after putting their kids in day-care, but Tara just couldn't see herself as one of them.

Tara lost her mother the year before and missed her terribly. They had been very close. Her mother had been an emotional support as Tara navigated motherhood. When Tara's husband traveled for work, her mother would come to provide another set of hands in the home. Now, Tara was left alone with the children, a mountain of grief, and a husband who traveled and was often unavailable. Feeling overwhelmed, she was beginning to resent his travel schedule. It kept him from taking an active role in child-rearing, and she didn't know how to tell him how overburdened she felt.

I knew Tara was grieving, possibly depressed, lonely, intellectually understimulated, and that she wanted more help from her husband with the kids.

As she finished telling her story, she asked, "What's wrong with me? I'm in my early thirties—I'm supposed to be at my sexual peak. But I've lost all interest in sex."

I suggested the better question for her to ask was not about sex, but about the rest of her life: "Why do I feel this way?"

P art I of this book provided an introduction to embodied sexuality. Part II is going to take you through the embodiment process. When women know what they like about sex and how to ask for it, we know they enjoy it more. This leads to sexual empowerment, which is a state we want you to achieve. But getting to that full empowerment is tricky when we don't have any framework for understanding or exploring what our individual authentic sexuality is and what might be in the way of harnessing it. The next two chapters are dedicated to that aim. They explore the different facets of what we call your *sexual core*, or the factors that make you who you are as a sexual being.

We'll start by introducing a biopsychosocial approach. This approach explains that a variety of factors impact who you are at your sexual core at any given time. We call these your external *influencers*, and they fall into four main categories: biological, psychological, interpersonal, and sociocultural. Your influencers work together to form a delicate balance; if any one particular area of your life is off-kilter, it upsets the equilibrium. Rather than seeing them as separate and boxed off from the other, think of the borders between each influencer as permeable. Each is part of the constantly changing and dynamic system. Understanding and addressing your influencers, therefore, is not a one-time thing; instead, it's a lifelong series of opportunities to connect with your sexuality.

Changes in your body, in the way you see the world, and in the people around you can affect the way you experience your sexual core. Change is constant, whether it be gradual, like going through menopause, or abrupt, such as the death of a family member or birth of a baby. Those life changes often bring on increased levels of stress. As Tara experienced, giving up her career and losing her mother, combined with the common physical and emotional stresses of parenting small children, had a direct effect on her desire to have sex with her husband.

If an influencer is red hot and flaring with dysfunction, disease, or stress, it will more than likely stop us in our tracks, demanding attention. The more subtle ones might not be hot enough to grab our attention, but they have an insidious way of diminishing our desire to engage with our sexuality.

Of course, it's unlikely that our life is ever in a perfect state of homeostasis. Life is life, and we're all doing the best we can to juggle all we've got twirling in the air. Things happen: we suffer a financial setback; fight with our partner; or out of nowhere, get sick with the worst cold ever. Remember, the boundary of each influencer is porous, so the four areas can spill over into each other. For example, if you break your leg and gain twenty pounds, both biological influencers, depression, a psychological influencer, might set in.

It is also important that we help you understand how influencers throughout your life affect your sexual expression. We invite you to explore the idea that it's also a two-way street. Just as the sexual core is impacted by the outside influencers, your sexual core can affect your influencers too. Expressing yourself sexually through pleasure, either on your own or with a partner, positively impacts the four factors of influence. The more sexual pleasure you experience, the better you feel physically (biology), the happier you are mentally (psychology), the more accepting you are of positive social values regarding sex (sociocultural), and quite frankly, the more fulfilling your relationships will be (interpersonal).

This chapter, therefore, will help you understand the complexity of your sexuality and help you identify what may have created roadblocks that have kept you from reaching your fullest sexual expression. By bringing the influencers more into balance, you increase the probability of feeling more sexual pleasure. Remember, pleasure itself can create more balance in the rest of your life, making a healthy relationship with sexuality a part of your overall well-being.

Biological Influencers

Let's begin by looking at some of the *biological influencers* that can affect your sexual core. We'll start with your hormones. They matter—a lot. You probably noticed this when you reached puberty and your sex hormones first came on board. Their arrival prompted changes in your body, such as the growth of pubic hair, increased breast tissue, and the onset of your first period. If you have ever been pregnant, you surely noticed major shifts throughout your pregnancy and after delivery. As your body moves through menopause, your hormones shift yet again, reversing many of the changes that were brought on by puberty.

Hormones are natural chemical substances produced by the endocrine system. They are secreted from glands throughout the body, including the pituitary, hypothalamus, thymus, adrenals, pancreas, thyroid, and for us women, our ovaries. Once released, they travel through the bloodstream, carrying messages to different cells in the body.

There are three main female sex hormones: *estrogen, progesterone*, and *testosterone*. Both estrogen and progesterone are present throughout the menstrual cycle, during which they take turns dominating the system. Just prior to menstruation, the levels of both hormones drop, often causing symptoms of premenstrual syndrome (PMS). All women have small amounts of testosterone. This surprises some people; we often think about testosterone solely as a male hormone, but it's crucial for women as well.

Estrogen primarily comes from the ovaries and increases between menstruation and ovulation. Estrogen is a group of sex steroid hormones, including *estrone, estriol,* and *estradiol.* Estrogen performs a multitude of tasks including but not limited to bone health, mental health, and pregnancy. It also helps keep the vaginal tissues healthy, moist and receptive to friction. Estrogen sharply decreases during menopause, which causes the vaginal dryness that many menopausal and postmenopausal women talk about. Some women experience painful *fissures*, or superficial tears in the tissue of the vulva and at the opening of the vagina, when their estrogen is low.

Progesterone begins to rise after ovulation and is often called the "pregnancy hormone." It helps build the uterine lining and is produced continuously throughout pregnancy. Like estrogen, progesterone is primarily produced by the ovaries. It's well known that progesterone has been linked to headaches, irregular menstruation, anxiety, and depression. Throughout a woman's menstrual years, progesterone and estrogen are in an intricate dance. Once a woman goes through menopause, that dance slows, significantly decreasing the production of both hormones.

It's important to note that hormonal birth control—whether taken orally, through a hormone-secreting IUD or ring, or via patch, implant, or injection—works to control that estrogen-progesterone cycling. We're both huge advocates of women's access to contraception and do not intend to knock it. That said, it's important to understand that the continual use of hormonal birth control affects hormones in a way that, for some women, also affects desire. And a lack of desire can lead to a lack of arousal, which—bingo!—can be the source of some women's sexual pain. In an ideal world, every woman would have both: an easy way to proactively control her fertility and hot, juicy, pain-free sex. That's why it's best to discuss your birth control options and their impact on your desire and arousal with your doctor or healthcare provider.

Testosterone affects reproductive and bone health in women and can have a positive impact on their desire for sex. Importantly, testosterone is readily converted to female sex hormones, including estrogens. At puberty, both boys and girls have an initial surge of both testosterone and estrogen that continues into young adulthood, contributing to breast development and voice changes. Naturally, as with the other sex hormones, testosterone levels decrease throughout the life cycle.

Other hormones, like *cortisol* and *serotonin*, affect sexual health indirectly by affecting our general well-being. *Cortisol* helps the body respond to stress. In high-stress situations, cortisol levels spike, giving us a natural energy boost to handle the situation. Like cortisol, *serotonin* has a strong hold on our mental health. It also regulates appetite and digestion, bone health, sex, and sleep.

And finally, let's look at *oxytocin*, another feel-good hormone associated with relaxation, empathy, trust, and psychological stability. Oxytocin is released during hugging and kissing. With sexual arousal, oxytocin levels increase, rising even more with orgasm.[43] It is often called the "love hormone," as it enhances bonding behavior and attachment between couples.

This was just a quick breakdown of the most important hormones that impact a woman's sexual core. Hormones aren't the only biological influencers that affect your sexual core. What you eat and drink matters too. Do you maintain a healthy and balanced diet that is specific to your needs across the life cycle? Do you have digestive issues? Are you well-hydrated?

What medications and over-the-counter supplements do you take? Many medications include sexual side effects listed in a tiny font. If you're taking medication and having trouble with desire, it may be worth it to check the fine print.

We always ask about bowel and bladder function, as much as it may surprise the women who come to see us. And we ask about sleep: what is your sleep pattern like? Do you feel well-rested or constantly fatigued? Substance use and misuse permeate our sexual core and diminish normal function, so we often ask about the role that recreational substances play in a woman's life. Other biological factors, such as cardiovascular and neurological health as well as acute or chronic disease and their treatment, do the same and warrant at least a cursory investigation.

Perhaps you have abdominal or genital scar tissue as a result of a physical injury or surgical procedure. Maybe you've been suffering with chronic pain located somewhere else on your body, other than your genitals. The very presence of chronic pain has a massive effect on your availability, willingness, and desire to be sexual.

The list goes on to include pelvic floor issues (birth trauma), painful menstrual cycles, and having a history of endometriosis. All of these biological factors impact women's optimal sexual health.

A Note from Dee:

Hormonal variability creates change throughout the female life cycle, beginning with puberty and menstruation, progressing through the childbearing years, and ending with menopause. All are normal and natural parts of life.

That said, we couldn't write a book about sex without discussing childbirth and its effects on desire. I'm not exactly sure who decided six weeks after delivery is the optimal time to wait before having sex, but that's the standard of care in the US. Women frequently come to me asking whether this is reasonable, and the answer is: well, it depends. The time it takes for a woman to be comfortable with sex varies from woman to woman. Many just aren't ready at that point; others are. Those who have a medically uneventful delivery typically recover more quickly than someone who undergoes a cesarean delivery or who tears with childbirth. As a general rule, no one should tell a woman when she should return to penetrative sex. The decision is all hers.

With rare exceptions, caring for newborns is exhausting. Day-to-day functions are difficult as time management becomes a thing of the past. Decreased estrogen, sleep deprivation, feeling as big as a moose, and worrying that you'll never want to have sex again can all cause acute depression. If not acknowledged and managed, depression, combined with hormonal factors, may progress to postpartum depression, which is a serious problem that needs to be addressed with your practitioner. Feeling sexy is often the last thing on your mind, especially at bedtime. Over time, you find that you have disconnected from yourself and your sensuality in lieu of caring for your precious and dependent baby.

Consider the biological influencers associated with pregnancy and childbirth. Throughout your pregnancy, your body—your pelvic floor and your abdominal muscles in particular—take on increasing stress as they support your growing baby. Physiologically, birth can cause trauma. If a vaginal birth includes an episiotomy or perineal tearing, your vulva needs to heal. Following a cesarean section, you need to recover from a routine, but major, abdominal surgery. Your body continues to change hormonally and physiologically following delivery as it prepares for feeding (whether you breastfeed or not), regains normal bowel and bladder function, and works to get strong again in the areas most stressed (pelvis, abdomen, and hips).

In any case, six weeks may not be enough to recover from all that. To further complicate things, we're instinctively wired (we are mammals, after all) to focus on caring for our helpless newborns, not *to seek out sex for pleasure—much less to conceive again. If you're breastfeeding, your oxytocin, which I like to think of as the "snuggle hormone," increases every few hours when you nurse, leading you to get your "snuggle on" with your baby rather than seeking out your partner. Though your estrogen levels soar during pregnancy, they tank follow-*

ing delivery and continue to stay low as long as you breastfeed. Running low on estrogen keeps your warning light on—your vulva and vagina are hormonally inhospitable (decreased mucous production, thinner walls) and your desire for sex is desperately low.

As hard as it is, be sure not to forget about YOU. Schedule time for yourself, however you can, and use it as time for you. Try to tap back into your sensuality—light a candle, turn on your favorite music, or schedule a massage. Start doing pelvic floor exercises, perhaps while you feed your baby. Reacquaint yourself with your vulva by getting out a mirror. Chances are things aren't nearly as bad as you might imagine. Welcome your clitoris back into your life slowly.

In the meantime, don't totally forget about your partner. Be sure to compassionately tell him how you feel about what's happening. Listen to his needs, whatever they are. Find loving ways to connect him with you and your baby. Fathers understandably feel helpless with newborns, especially those who are nursed. Discuss ways to help him be a part of the process. The more connected he feels to what's going on, the more he will be able to empathize with what's happening and, with his support, the sooner you'll get back in the swing both physically and emotionally.

Finally, if you had trouble conceiving, I'll guess that sex became a mechanical, routine, and scheduled task. And if in vitro fertilization (IVF) *was required, the entire process may have been traumatic. Studies have shown that many women experience vulvar pain while some men become impotent during IVF due to the stress, pressure, and struggles. Respect that process and get counseling if possible. Trust me, you can get back to your norm. Be patient and compassionate with both yourself and your partner, and you will get through this.*

Bottom line? You need to be ready and interested in returning to penetrative sex before you attempt it. So go after any and all desire you feel and have fun experimenting with foreplay. Chances are you and your partner will be messing around one night, and you'll get so aroused you have an orgasm, and then penetration just happens!

Psychological Influencers

In the first part of this book, we discussed how all too often people feel some degree of shame around their sexuality. And to some extent, we explained why uncovering and addressing shame is so important. Now, let's look at it as one of the major *psychological influencers* impacting your sexual core.

We need to help you understand the difference between shame and guilt, as they are often mistakenly used interchangeably. *Shame* is a feeling that *we* are inherently wrong or bad. It is a feeling we have about *ourselves:* "I am bad. I am wrong." *Guilt* is a feeling of discomfort about *something we have or haven't done*. It is a feeling we have about *our behavior*, not ourselves: "I did something bad and I'm feeling guilty about it." The feeling states are different: I've done something wrong (guilt) versus I am wrong (shame). If either one resides inside of you, it will affect your sexual core.

Both shame and guilt decrease self-esteem. Women come to us feeling shame about their sexual histories and desires. Some women tell us they are bad because they had sex before marriage. Other women tell us they are wrong for wanting sex four times a week. Dee has heard far too often that a woman with chronic pain must have done something bad or wrong to cause the pain she is in: "I am bad. My mother told me not to use tampons and I did it anyway." In each case, the women expressed feelings (shame) about themselves, not their behavior. The reason shame is inherently more damaging is that it is internalized and deeply connected to our sense of ourselves. Guilt is more adaptive and more easily resolved. For instance, if you begin to exercise because you feel guilty for not doing so, your guilt wanes.

It is important to note any negative feelings you have about sex and sexuality. Were you given negative messages about flirting or being sexual? If so, do you hold any negative thoughts that cause you shame or guilt for having done so? These might include feeling bad for watching porn or for touching yourself at an early age because it felt good. What if you got caught enjoying either activity? Enjoying anything considered taboo or forbidden can also lead to feeling sexual shame.

Unwanted pregnancies, secret abortions, or suffering a miscarriage can deeply touch a woman at her sexual core. Many women are able to recover and heal from these events, whereas others struggle for the rest of their lives managing their sorrow.

There are other psychological influencers that can bring the sexual core out of balance; consider, for instance, the presence of psychiatric or mood disorders. In a great twist of irony, the most common set of drugs that the medical community uses to combat depression, *selective serotonin reuptake inhibitors (SSRIs)*, frequently have a libido-reducing side effect. This is an example of where a psychological influencer (depression) intersects with a biological intervention (medication). Both impact the sexual core.

What is the state of your overall mental health? Do you see the glass half-empty or is it half-full? How often do you experience happiness and joy? It might be that you find yourself barely surviving, feeling quite numb. What about anxiety and levels of high stress? These count too. In general, how do you feel about yourself? Are you confident, or is your self-esteem lagging?

A Note from Elizabeth:

I can't stress enough the importance of healthy self-esteem. Wearing confidence on your sleeve is attractive. It's important to believe that we're inherently good, doing our best, that we're offering something of value to the world, and that people like having us around. Self-esteem plays a big part in how we move through the world sexually too.

Let's take a look at one particular aspect of self-esteem that commonly influences women's sexual core: body image. When we're down about a bad hair day, how we smell, our age, our shape, or our size, it's hard to feel super turned on or sexy.

I used to ask my clients what they like and dislike about their bodies, and I was struck by how often the list of dislikes towered over their list of likes—as if in order to say anything positive about their bodies, they had to apologize for themselves. Eventually, I stopped asking for their dislikes, sticking to a simple list of likes instead. Some women found it hard to even come up with three things, but many really relished in the opportunity to tell me everything they loved, from the curve of their calves to the smoothness of their skin to their majestic height.

For example, I'll share with you a few things I like about myself: I love how tall I am. I love how bright and shiny my eyes are. I love my long, strong legs, which gracefully carry me down the ski slopes…well, most of the time! I love the way this body carries me through waves and waves of pleasure!

There's a whole world out there telling us we're not pretty enough, we don't wear the right clothes, or that "better" women are the ones who are more deserving of greater sex lives. Such messages bombard women daily. Given the onslaught of negative messaging and advertisements offering the latest innovations preying on female insecurities, it really is a revolutionary act to stand against these messages in a place of self-love and appreciation. This action has a massive and immediate impact on our ability to access our pleasure. It starts with you!

In addition, when a woman comes to us with low desire, we ask about any history of trauma. We simply cannot oversimplify a woman's experience of trauma. In the field of psychology, there are two kinds of trauma: large "T" traumas and small "t" traumas. Both result in heightened amounts of distress and decreased quality of life. Traumatic experiences often have the greatest negative overall effect on our sexual core. Rape, sexual and physical assault or abuse, incest, sexual harassment, and psychological abuse are of course the most extreme examples of this. It is important to point your attention to other, less obvious triggers for sexual trauma: choosing to have sex you don't want to have, being rejected by a lover, or even faking an orgasm. Though these events may seem less impactful, they can certainly land in the psyche as trauma and reduce your ability to access your sexuality later.

This is particularly true of early sexual experiences. When women come to us with pain, we often want to know about her first sexual experience, whether it was wanted or unwanted, pain-free or painful, and how she felt about it. This is because women often carry the trauma of their first sexual experience with them for a long time.

It often takes tremendous work to overcome such experiences and recreate a positive and healthy relationship with our body after experiencing trauma. This type of work is best done under the guidance of a trusted practitioner and can take quite some time. There are highly trained trauma therapists out there who work specifically with these issues. And the truth is, *we simply can't tackle emotional trauma full-on in this book because that is not our area of expertise.* But we do encourage you to get help if anything in this part of the chapter has struck a chord with you. Address the psychological aspects impacting your sexual core; don't let them linger in your system. Seek the help and guidance necessary for your healing so you can recover from the trauma and begin to explore pleasure. We believe, without a doubt, that you are worth it.

Interpersonal Influencers

If you're partnered, who you are at your sexual core is deeply affected by the level of general satisfaction in the relationship you have with your partner or spouse. One of the first questions we ask when partnered women come to work with us is: how is your relationship? Then we get specific: what's your home life like? What roles do each of you hold within the household, and how do you balance the workload? Do you and your spouse argue? Has there been an affair? Are there resentments that have built up over time that have yet to be resolved? Are they resolvable? Are you suffering but staying together for the kids? Do you feel safe to share your feelings, concerns, and desires with your partner? What is the quality of communication in your relationship? A woman's answers to these questions is very helpful in understanding what interpersonal factors may be impacting her ability and/or willingness to be sexual.

We ascertain the health of the relationship in myriad ways. Quality and frequency of sex is often a good barometer used to assess the health of a relationship. It is important to note when things change for a couple in the bedroom. If possible, we ask the couple to explore together when and why the change occurred. If problems in the relationship result in a decreased desire for sex, we suggest the couple work together to resolve the factor(s) impacting their sex life. Couples counseling is a great idea and solution that can help a couple get back on track.

When in a partnership that includes sexuality, it's important to consider another topic: what about your partner's physical and emotional health? Because this is a holistic approach, determining how your partner's biopsychosocial influencers may impact your own is a worthwhile exploration. Is he physically and emotionally balanced? What is his part in the health of your relationship? Does he have a social support system outside of you and your extended family, if you have one? His health and well-being are directly linked to your ability to engage and enjoy partnered sex.

In Part III of this book, we'll dive into partnered practices to help build intimacy as you work with your partner and (re)connect to your sexuality with reduced pain. The techniques and exercises we prescribe are universal and can be helpful in any relationship. But just as with trauma, we can't cover everything between these pages. If you're still struggling in your relationship after using our prescriptions, we recommend that you seek support from a therapist or counselor.

The interpersonal section of the sexual core also includes much more than the intimate relationship you have with your spouse or partner. It also includes relationships with friends and family. This is why we often ask women who are struggling to connect sexually about the strength of their friendships and other social ties.

In the case of Tara, whom you met at the beginning of this chapter, many of her relationships were work-related. When she chose to stay at home with her kids, she was cut off from that network and circle of friends. Isolated from her former colleagues and finding it difficult to connect with other stay-at-home moms, Tara was just plain lonely. She desperately wanted to return to her career, in part because she felt she would have more intellectually stimulating daily interactions by doing so. It's also worth noting Tara's grief. Her heart was heavy after losing her mother. She was also grieving the loss of her mother's love and support in raising her kids.

Helping Tara address the lack of meaningful connections in her social life and find fulfillment in her friends and family sphere were made part of her work. Improving the quality of communication with her husband was another critical piece needed to improve her overall sense of life satisfaction, which would, in turn, have an impact on her sexual core. Working with a grief counselor was also included in her individual prescription. All of these are interpersonal influencers.

Sociocultural Influencers

Lastly, we'll address the social and cultural factors that can impact a woman's sexual core. Factors such as when you were born (in the 1960s or 2000s?) and where you were raised (in a more socially progressive or more conservative area?) can have huge effects on how you see yourself, your sexuality, and your relationship to it. The beliefs and values you developed over the course of your lifetime, addressing such things as aging, menopause, and sex, all help to determine who you are as a woman. What culture did you grow up in, and how did that influence your belief system? Were you given a basic education about sex? If so, was it pleasure-based and comprehensive, or were you taught an abstinence-only or disease and pregnancy prevention curriculum? If you didn't receive formal education about sex, from whom did you learn about it—from other children, adults, television/media, direct experience, or some combination of the above?

Tara's decision to stop working—a great choice for many women, but not necessarily the best choice for her—was largely affected by these sociocultural influencers. Consciously or subconsciously, Tara internalized the message that "good moms stay at home with their kids." And that message was making her miserable.

Other examples of sociocultural influencers are spirituality and religion. You may be familiar with the Madonna/whore complex, wherein women are separated into two categories: those who are "pure," and those who are "not." Though many religions show some level of reverence to mothers, very few value or promote women's sexual pleasure. Whether we adopted these values or not, nearly all of us were raised in cultures that were somehow affected by this dichotomy. We want to be clear that religion itself is not the problem; it is entirely possible to be an advocate of and practice pleasure-forward sexuality and either be religious or hold strong spiritual beliefs. Rather, the issue is whether an empowered understanding of women's sexuality can fit into your understanding of the spiritual world that speaks to you.

Finally, when considering sociocultural influencers, it is important to consider your mother's sexual history, experiences, and beliefs. Many of us were raised by mothers who were shut down around their own sexuality. If this is your case, you may have subconsciously adopted her beliefs as your own. It's important to understand that throughout time, women have suffered from distorted viewpoints on female sexuality. The point is not to blame our mothers, other women, religion, or the culture around us. Let's heal these wounds and make the changes within ourselves so that we can better access our sexuality. As mothers, aunt, sisters, and friends, we can try to do better for our daughters *and* our sons by teaching them how to value and celebrate female sexuality in their own lives.

The following exercise will help you understand what's affecting your sexual core by considering the biological, psychological, interpersonal, and sociocultural influencers that are present in your life today.

Prescription 8

What's Influencing Your Sexual Core?

Some of the influencers affecting our sexual core cannot be changed, while others can. It's up to you to decide what aspects of your life you are able to shift, as well as what, if anything, you *want* to shift. To get started, it's useful to take an inventory of the influencers affecting your sexual core, both positively and negatively. This exercise will help you do precisely that.

This chapter includes only one prescription—but it's a big one, and we expect it to take quite some time. You'll make four lists in your journal. Take the time to quietly reflect on each of them. Reread the sections above as they provide examples of factors that might have impacted your ability to fully experience your sexuality. If there's something we've missed (most likely we have), make sure to include it on your paper. You can do this all at once or in several chunks of time. As you write, remember that it's normal for influencers in one category to spill over to another, so don't be concerned if you don't know where a certain item goes; just list it twice.

We hope that by now, you understand that your influencers are dynamic—they're always changing. Whenever you feel yourself losing touch with pleasure over the course of your life, you can return to this prescription to see what's changed and how each set of influencers may be affecting who you are at your sexual core.

What You'll Need:

- Forty-plus minutes of relative privacy, potentially split into four ten-minute segments.

- A journal and a pen.

- Optional: Extra paper.

Let's Get Started!

- Start with your biological influencers. Ask yourself: What is your overall state of health? Do you have chronic illnesses? Are you menstruating, and if so, how is your cycle? If not, are you still in the menopausal process, or is the process complete? Do you have injuries? What is your diet like? Do you get enough sleep and exercise? What medications and hormones are you on? List all the biological factors influencing your sexual core.

- Move on to your psychological influencers. Do you suffer from anxiety or depression? How is your self-esteem? Do you harbor shame around sex? Do you feel that you deserve pleasure? List all the psychological factors influencing your sexual core.

- Move on to your sociocultural influencers. What kind of sex education did you receive (if any)? How were you parented? What beliefs did you inherit from your upbringing? Which societal "norms" did you embrace, and which did you toss away? What are your cultural and/ or religious beliefs about sex? List all the sociocultural factors influencing your sexual core.

- Move on to your interpersonal influencers. If you are currently in a relationship, what is it like? Do you and your partner communicate well? How do you disagree? What are your schedules like? Do you feel that the responsibilities are distributed fairly between you? Are you attracted to your partner? What is the state of your partner's physical and emotional health? Is your partner sexually available? Who else are you close to in your life? How might your relationships with those people be affecting you? List all the interpersonal factors influencing your sexual core.

- Once you have completed the exercise, look at the lists you made pertaining to each influencer. Understand that these lists are dynamic; they provide a unique snapshot of this moment in time, and they will change.

- Now, is there anything in your list that you want to change? If so, circle it and make a commitment to yourself to shift this area of your life for the sake of your sexual pleasure.

- Finally, is there anything in your list that you cannot change and will have to accept? If so, underline it and make a commitment to yourself to accept it for the sake of your sexual pleasure.

- Take a moment to look at your paper one final time before putting it away. Remember, you can do this exercise again any time you like—it will always be different!

Taking a Look at Your Own Life

In this chapter, you learned that your sexual core is affected by the biological, psychological, interpersonal, and sociocultural influencers that surround it. In Tara's case, her ability to access her sexuality was blocked by some of these influencers. Dee's prescriptions, therefore, all focused around addressing the factors in Tara's life that she could control. It was a start to helping her regain connection with herself as a sexual being and rebuild her self-esteem.

In the next chapter, we'll explore the internal aspects of your sexual core. As sexual beings, we are as diverse as the rocks in a riverbed, each one of us unique and absolutely beautiful. The more we know ourselves, the better we can express ourselves, opening the doors to deeper and deeper pleasure. Read on to learn how you can understand the internal aspects of your sexual core. It's part of the greater pleasure prescription we offer: The one that helps us become enthusiastic, empowered sexual beings.

CHAPTER SIX

Identifying Your Sexual Core

A Note from Elizabeth:

Sarah always felt positive about sex and her sexual experiences. She had one long-term boyfriend for most of her twenties, and sex with him had been great, although she didn't orgasm that often. Now in her early thirties, Sarah was seeing a new guy who she really liked. At first, sex with him seemed to be going well. But he had experienced different types of sex with more partners which left her feeling self-conscious about meeting his expectations. Sarah realized that he was much better at asking for what he wanted; she, on the other hand, often had no idea how her turn-on happened.

I asked Sarah about her self-pleasuring habits, and she quickly responded that she had been self-pleasuring for many years. It typically took her more than twenty minutes to climax, which she described as "way too long." She was concerned that she didn't think about sex with the new beau "enough." In part, this was because it was hard for her to reach orgasm while having sex with someone else. Watching porn and self-pleasuring was just easier.

But the porn itself was bothering her too. She enjoyed touching her vulva but had only recently seen it up close using a mirror. Sarah had fleshy, asymmetrical inner lips. Suddenly, Sarah had realized that she didn't look like any of the women she'd seen on screen. This made it harder to enjoy receiving oral sex, something she had always loved in the past. Sarah had heard that vulvas could be surgically altered and asked what I thought about it.

She also wanted help with her relationship in general. She liked her boyfriend, as did all of her friends. But his experience level was intimidating, and honestly, it wasn't making their sex better for her. It seemed like they were each turned on by different things. Sarah felt like she and her first boyfriend had naturally been "a perfect match, like two puzzle pieces that fit together" both physically and emotionally. Would she ever find such a perfect match again?

After our first meeting, I looked over the notes I had taken. Phrases like "doesn't know who she is" and "doesn't know what she wants" peppered the page. I saw her relationship with her first boyfriend as a positive one—easy and everything flowed until it no longer worked. What she needed now was to learn about herself with and through her new partner. My job was to help Sarah learn the size and shape of her own puzzle piece to further explore compatibility with her new partner. It was about helping Sarah discover who she was as a sexual being and finding her unique way of expressing it with her new partner.

Part of Sarah's challenge was that she didn't really know what turned her on or how she wanted to express her sexuality. She began to question her unique anatomy and how it looked and functioned, was concerned about her arousal pattern, and felt incompatible with her current boyfriend. What turned him on seemed foreign to her. Though she was sure she was better matched with her previous boyfriend, she didn't know exactly *how* or *why* that was the case.

In this chapter, we will describe what helped Sarah understand the shape of her puzzle piece. As we move deeper into the chapter, you'll be invited to do the same. There's so much to learn about who you are as a sexual being! And it inherently involves understanding the wide variations in human sexuality. There are so many ways to be—so many anatomical types, so many styles of turn-on, so many forms of healthy sexual expression—and they're all okay.

Together, these make up the internal aspects of your sexual core. They include your unique anatomy, how and when you get turned on, and how you enjoy expressing that turn-on. Like your external influencers, your internal aspects can change over time, but not nearly as easily or rapidly.

During one of the episodes of the Showtime hit series *Masters of Sex*, the character Dr. William Masters asked, "How can something deviate when there is no norm? Why would we expect two humans to express their sexuality in the same way? Your body is as particular and individualistic as a kiss. Where there is such infinite variety, there is no norm, only deviation."[44]

And it's true. When it comes to variations in anatomy, the only norm is diversity. Let's consider variations in the color of vulvas. As we mentioned in Chapter One, women with darker skin are as likely to have pinkish vulvas as they are to have dark ones, while women with lighter skin can sport rich purple and brown hues just as easily as rosy, beige, or mauve. No two vulvas or vaginas are exactly alike, just as no two people are. Their size, shape, and color are as diverse as we are. And they're often diverse even within themselves; labia size can differ from left to right, just like our feet and breasts are slightly different sizes, and a single vulva can display a range of beautiful colors. It's not enough to say that vulvar diversity is normal; it's *the norm.*

We'll look at how this diversity has been categorized in the sexual practices of Quodoushka. Though the teachings of Quodoushka are extensive, we offer you just a taste to help you see how your specific vulva shape and size can reveal the types of pleasure you may enjoy the most.

Next, we'll discuss diversity in terms of turn-on. You'll learn how to address any discord between your physical and psychological turn on. Then we'll introduce the Erotic Blueprint™ Types, a system that can help you create deeper connection and sexual satisfaction. Knowing which of the five types ignites your arousal will help you express your sexual needs more clearly so they can be satisfied more often.

Finally, we'll discuss many forms and ways for you to share your sexuality with others. We live in a culture that exalts certain forms of sexual expression over others. This can give the false impression that there's one "normal" way to relate to sexuality, and that everything else is somehow wrong. But this is simply not the case. Sexual expression is a form of creative expression, and the range of possibilities is both wide and deep.

As you read, pay attention to what resonates. Just as you cataloged the external influencers affecting your sexual core in the previous chapter, catalog the descriptors that hit home for you in this one. Then, at the end of the chapter, use the prescriptions that Elizabeth offered Sarah to help find the internal aspects of your authentic sexual self.

Your Unique Anatomy

At the beginning of this book, you learned about the female arousal network and the anatomy of your vulva. You're well-versed now, knowing no two vulvas are alike. As you've progressed through the prescriptions in this book, looking at your vulva up close and exploring self-pleasure, you've come to understand a little more about what makes your vulva unique.

We hope you are able to see your unique anatomy as normal and beautiful. We've stated this before, but we want to be very clear that asymmetry, a wide hue of colors, and clitoral hood and lip size differences are all normal. As doctor and yoga teacher Wendy Zerin, MD, says, "Symmetry is an external aesthetic construct which bears little relationship to the reality of the body."[45] It's very important to understand this because, today, many medical professionals are asked, "Am I normal?"

Disturbingly, a growing number of medical providers answer this question by recommending labiaplasty, a procedure that reshapes and /or reduces the size of the labia. The labial tissue that is cut and removed is filled with nerve endings and blood vessels and is part of the erectile network that contributes to feeling sexual pleasure. It's important to remember that when any part of the body is cut, scar tissue forms, reducing sensation. And, when we're talking about the labia, it's no different. Scar tissue that forms following surgery to this highly sensitive area can cause a loss of sensation and pleasure.

The very idea of labiaplasty infuriates us as professionals and as women. It is, however, a woman's personal choice. We must stress the need to be well-informed before deciding to undergo the procedure. Women's sexual health professionals and associations are against this particular cosmetic surgery. Many medical associations have come out against the procedure meant to "fix" a woman's discomfort with her genital appearance, posting position papers on the first page of their websites. Furthermore, the idea that labiaplasty exists reinforces the idea that there's just *something wrong* with some women's labia—an idea we wholeheartedly reject.

A Note from Elizabeth:

I am lucky to have three wonderful sisters. As I stated in Chapter One, like Sarah, I have large inner labia. At some point in my journey toward accepting my beautiful labia, I began to wonder whether my sisters had labia that looked like mine. After all, even though we have the same mother and father, our noses, eyes, and mouths don't look alike. What about our vulvas?

I had only contemplated this in passing, never imaging a way I would find out. Almost out of nowhere an opportunity presented itself the day of my spectacular wedding. For the event, I wore a big, heavy wedding dress that prevented me from going to the toilet unassisted. As I had held my sister Margaret's dress on her wedding day, she was the one who helped lift mine while I hovered over the loo to do my business. With Margaret underneath my dress, it suddenly came to mind that here was my one chance, so I asked, "Do your lips look like mine?"

Her response was classic. "No, you can wear red lipsticks. I have to wear more pinkish tones."

I bopped her on the head and said, "Not those lips. I'm wondering about your lower ones."

My sister emerged from under my skirt with a shocked look on her face. She paused and asked, "Um, where's this going?"

At my urging, she left to get our other sisters as I wanted to do a "show and tell." When she returned with only one, I shoved the two of them into the oversized bathroom stall, wondering if our vulvas looked at all alike. I said, "If I show you mine, will your show me yours?" Here's where a wee bit of vodka helped my quest; all three of us were just tipsy enough to venture further.

With the help of a cell phone flashlight, we hiked up our dresses and each looked at the others. What we saw was fantastic. Our vulvas didn't look at all alike! And each vulva was undoubtedly, uniquely beautiful!

Vulvar diversity is not new information. As early as 400 BCE, classical Indian texts referred to different-sized *yonis* (the Hindi word for *vulva*) and divided women into three categories—gazelles, mares, and elephants—according to the characteristics of her vulva. Each was equally revered.[46] In *The Perfumed Garden,* a fifteenth-century sex manual written in Arabic, author Sheikh Nefzawi lists dozens of names to categorize the female genitals, including *the yearning one, the voluptuous, the watering can, the long one, the deep one, the one with a little nose,* and the particularly delightful *the one that swells* (hello, clitoral engorgement!). The author goes on to describe others as *the delicious one, the juicy,* and, simply, *the beautiful.*[47]

More recent drawings and descriptions were published during the twentieth century. As you saw way back in Chapter One, in order to counterbalance that generic textbook vulva, we included the beautiful illustrations that Robert Dickinson published in 1933. Dickinson eventually concluded that "Here, as in other regions, one learns to ask, not what is 'average' or 'normal' but rather 'what is the most common dimension or grouping?'"[48] In 1974, sex educator Betty Dodson released the drawings she had made of her girlfriends in her groundbreaking book, *Sex for One.* These drawings beautifully depicted a wide range of vulvas.[49]

But for us, the most useful system of understanding vulvar diversity comes from specific knowledge passed down through the generations by the Twisted Hairs Nagual Elders of the Sweet Medicine Sundance Path. These teachings are known as the sexual practices of Quodoushka and have been described by Amara Charles in her book, *The Sexual Practices of Quodoushka.*[50] The teachings utilize a deliberate classification system that identifies nine female and male genital anatomy types and how each differs in the ways it likes to be stimulated to achieve arousal and experience pleasure. Since our focus is on vulvas, here we'll focus solely on women's genitalia.

The nine types of female genitalia take measurements of both the vulva and the vagina into account. The external characteristics of the vulva are generally understood based on the following: the size and contour of the labia (both inner and outer), the distance between the clitoris and the vaginal opening (measured with the woman's own fingers placed sideways, with her fingertips pointing toward one thigh—some have room to place one or two fingers, while others have room for three or four), the shape of the clitoral hood, and the general size and shape of the vulva as a whole. Internally, Quodoushka considers the size of the vagina itself (both depth and width) and the location of the G-spot, as some are close to the opening of the vagina, while others are deeper along the vaginal wall. The importance of this structural difference is quite significant for women because when various erotic zones are clustered close together, a woman tends to reach orgasms much more quickly, whereas when they are farther apart, her erogenous zones may not be as easily stimulated all at once. This is only one of the many ways the structure of our genital anatomy influences our lovemaking. The system also considers other measures such as the amount of lubrication produced, its taste, and the average length of time it takes the woman to reach orgasm.

To help you understand the anatomy types better, we will look at four of the most distinct types. They are the four that sit in what's known as the cardinal directions—north, east, south, and west—based on a Native American medicine wheel. Four more sit in between the cardinal points—northwest, southwest, northeast, and southeast—and display qualities from the two directions they sit in between. The ninth type occupies the center of the medicine wheel and possesses qualities alternatively from each of the other directions. We will only cover the four cardinal points in this book.

What we find so appealing and useful is that because Quodoushka presents the four directions, the four elements—wind, fire, water, and earth—and assigns an animal totem to each nine of the vulvar types, this system is the most practical, uplifting, and empowering set of teachings we have found. Discovering the uniqueness of each type has helped countless women cast away shame and find the real beauty of their vulvas so that they can enjoy sexual intimacy way more often.

When asked specifically about the use of animal names, Amara Charles told us this:

It never ceases to amaze me how brilliantly indigenous people correlated various characteristics of certain animals to discern specific patterns of arousal that define the traits of each genital anatomy type. Perhaps it was their keen tracking and hunting abilities and living so closely attuned to nature that led them to choose these particular animal names. If you consider the differences in style between how a buffalo saunters and then stampedes across the plains, how a wolf's howl carries into the dark night, how deer gracefully nibble the leaves and then swiftly dash away or how sheep like to nudge and stay quite close to one another, you can begin to imagine the very different temperaments of each sexual anatomy type. Perhaps what is most remarkable is just how accurately these animal names help to describe fascinating differences in both the physiological erotic structure of our genitals and the kinds of approaches to sexual arousal we tend to like best as lovers.[51]

Before we go further, it's important to state that while you may recognize yourself in one of the following descriptions, we are only providing a shortened version of a much larger and greater teaching. Attending a Quodoushka workshop will be of most benefit to those who are interested in learning more about their specific anatomy type and the system as a piece of the whole Quodoushka teaching.

With that said, we'll talk about the first of the four types we are describing:

The Sheep Vulva

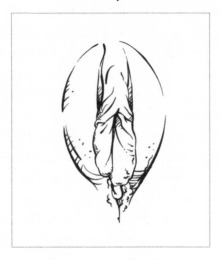

Image copyrighted and reprinted with permission of Amara Charles

The most noticeable thing about this vulva is the long hood that forms a tunnel covering the clitoris. This vulva is puffy, almost rounded. Sheep Women tend to have rather long vaginal canals and can enjoy extended, deep penetration. Due to their abundant labial tissue and long clitoral hood, they tend to like oral sex even more. Their long hood has been described as part of their superpower; sucking and stroking it can evoke intense pleasure. Their inner labia are fairly thin. When stimulated, a Sheep Woman produces generous amounts of vaginal secretions, which is why these women, more often than not, aren't the ones reaching for the lube. Their vaginal secretions often taste sweet. A Sheep Woman is described as watery, teary, and emotionally sensitive. She needs a heartfelt connection for sex to be meaningful to her. The distance between her glans and vaginal opening is between two to three of her fingers laid horizontally.

The Buffalo Vulva

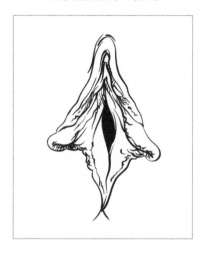

Image copyrighted and reprinted with permission of Amara Charles

You may remember Elizabeth's note about her experience as a Buffalo Woman from Chapter One. Elizabeth was terribly embarrassed by the size and shape of her vulva. Her labia were a source of emotional pain for her, which is a pain that is shared by many other women with the labia of a Buffalo Woman prior to learning these teachings. The Buffalo vulva has large, thick inner labia that protrude from the outer labia, curling and hanging downward. *Rugose*, or having many wrinkles, is a great way to describe the inner labia of the Buffalo Woman. In the nooks and crannies of the Buffalo lips, bits of toilet paper seem to land and stay behind. Despite this, part of a Buffalo woman's superpower can come from her abundant anatomy. There's great pleasure to be had having these large lips stroked, licked, and sucked. When compared to the other anatomy types, the Buffalo Woman has a shallower vagina, though its entrance is wide. The in-and-out motion of vaginal penetration itself is often incredibly enjoyable for her. Penetrating a Buffalo Woman deeply, however, can initially cause pain if she and her partner don't take care to find the right depth or position. With increased arousal, she can accommodate deeper penetration. The Buffalo Woman produces moderate amounts of salty- or earthy-tasting lubricant. Reaching climax generally takes longer for a Buffalo Woman; her arousal cycle is normally about fifteen to twenty minutes on average. She likes being in a state of extended arousal, which could last for days (another superpower), and she really enjoys taking things slowly. Like the Sheep Woman, the Buffalo Woman can usually fit two to three fingers between her clitoral glans and her vaginal opening.

The Wolf Vulva

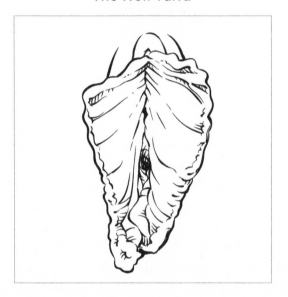

Image copyrighted and reprinted with permission of Amara Charles

The first thing to notice about the Wolf Woman is the shape and thinness of her inner labia, which can resemble butterfly wings once they are spread open and apart. These lips are smooth and thin, and often, one of them is larger than the other. Her hood covers the clitoris but usually isn't much larger than that. The Wolf Woman spends a lot of time in her head, has a rich fantasy life, but has a harder time getting into her body than the other anatomy types. Wolf Women have reported that they enjoy having penetrative intercourse while they are on their menstrual cycles. Because of their distinct vulva shape and size, they may particularly enjoy strong oral and clitoral stimulation, they tend to be wet, and generally taste salty-sweet. They have a natural proclivity to make noise during lovemaking—think *howling at the moon!* Social conditioning, however, may have caused them to suppress such vocal expression. If a Wolf Woman can let go of that, her growls, grunts, and groans add to the pleasure of the experience. Her arousal cycle, generally speaking, is about ten to fifteen minutes before reaching orgasm. (As a reminder, timing differences are simply differences. Nothing is good or bad, right or wrong—just different.) The Wolf Woman can usually fit one to two fingers between her clitoral glans and her vaginal opening.

The Deer Vulva

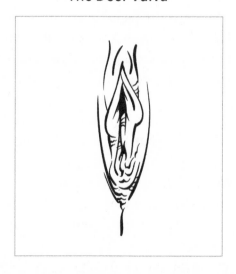

Image copyrighted and reprinted with permission of Amara Charles

The Deer Woman is immediately characterized by her overall petite vulva. Her outer labia are thin, her inner labia are small, and the entire vulva can be less than an inch from top to bottom. Deer Women get a lot of clitoral stimulation from penetration because their barely hooded glans is usually just a finger or less from the vaginal opening, meaning reaching orgasm can be quick and fairly easy. Because of the short distance between her clitoris and vaginal opening, a Deer Woman may be more likely than other anatomy types to orgasm from vaginal penetration alone. Many Deer Women are able to have multiple orgasms. Their orgasms are what all other orgasms are unfairly measured against. We've been conditioned to believe if we don't orgasm quickly and in multiple succession, we're not sexy, we're frigid, or we're broken. Deer Women tend to be quite dry with minimal natural lubrication; these women have packets of lube in their nightstands, their glove compartments, backpacks, and purses. What natural lube they do produce has a sweet-tart taste. It's important to note that many women believe their vulvas should look like a Deer Woman's because this is the type of vulva we've been conditioned to expect; they are the vulvas that are depicted most often in porn due to their petite size and shape. Remember how we stated in Chapter One that most porn actresses and nude models are chosen for the shape of their anatomy? Most photographic images of vulvas that do not look like a Deer Woman's vulva have been digitally altered to do so. This often affects women's expectations for their own vulvas.

Perhaps you've seen yourself in one of these images or read one of the four description that make you think, "Hey, I might be a _____ Woman." There is so much more to the Quodoushka teachings specific to female anatomy types. We've offered you just a taste here and hope we've piqued your interest to study more.[52]

When Arousal and Turn-On Don't Align

Just like your anatomy is unique, so too is your turn-on. There's a wide range of what turns a person on, both physically and psychologically. Ideally, these work in tandem. But sometimes, physical and psychological turn-on simply don't align. When this is the case, and when turn-on has been challenging to access for any reason (be it physical pain or anything else), we suggest tapping into your turn-on wherever it comes a-knocking. Whatever turns you on, even just a little bit, follow it. It will help you understand more about your sexual core.

A Note from Dee:

In truth, researchers don't really know for certain how arousal and desire interact in women. For instance, some women's bodies can be turned on, producing physical symptoms of arousal such as tingling and swelling in the vulva, without their brains fully realizing what is happening. And other women have a psychological desire to be sexual, but their bodies don't respond physically—there's no lubrication, no increased blood flow, etc. In Emily Nagoski's book, Come as You Are, *she coins the phrase* arousal noncondordance *to describe any discord between psychological and physical arousal.[53] In contrast, the medical system's current diagnostic criteria describes a lack of concordance between physiological and psychological arousal as* sexual interest/arousal disorder (SIAD). *We find this name to be unfortunate because the diagnosis does not exactly describe what's happening for these women.*

Lest we jump to conclusions, it's important to notice that the science suggests this isn't just an issue of the disconnect we discussed in Part I of this book. A recent paper suggests that women with arousal and desire difficulties are actually more *aware than other women of what's happening in their bodies.[54] For the first time, we're considering the possibility that physiological arousal may precede psychological desire, contrary to what our entire society has thought in the past. But these results aren't conclusive. It may be that there is no one direction for arousal to spread—that some women will start with physiological arousal and develop psychological desire from there, while others may move in the opposite direction.*

We need more research in this area—much more. I can't stress this enough. Recently, I read a study that mentioned how "Female sexual function is under-studied, and mechanisms of clitoral engorgement-relaxation are incompletely understood."[55] I agree; we need more of everything in terms of women's sexual pleasure.

In the meantime, keep track of your own turn-on, tapping into what makes you tick as a sexual being. As we've shown you throughout the book, there are a lot of benefits to doing so; by becoming the master of your own sexual functioning, you can learn a whole lot about yourself.

Your Erotic Blueprint Type

Humans are turned on by a variety of things. Here, we'll present a brilliant system developed by Certified Somatic Sex Educator and sexologist Jaiya of Jaiya, Inc. The system was designed to help you understand your individual Erotic Blueprint™ Type so you can create deeper connection and greater sexual satisfaction. You may be familiar with Gary Chapman's *The Five Love Languages*. Jaiya created a similar tool, but one that describes five ways we source our arousal and turn-on, or what she calls the *Erotic Blueprint™ Types*. Each one of them is like a specific key that opens a doorway to a distinct style of turn-on. The Erotic Blueprints™ are access points to your turn-on and arousal. Knowing which of the five types ignites your arousal will help you express your sexual needs more clearly, which will result in them being satisfied more often.

When we follow our turn-on, whenever and however we feel it, we start to connect more to our sexuality. Notice the variety of things that turn you on. There's great benefit knowing that what turns you on may be different from what turns someone else on. Each one of us is wired differently for pleasure. When exploring this, it is extremely helpful to identify what kinds of things we're excited by and those that, quite frankly, seem to turn us off.

Armed with the language of the Erotic Blueprints, you will be able to express more clearly and specifically what lights your fire and what extinguishes it in a blink of an eye. The Erotic Blueprints are about where we each source our turn-on. They are meant to help create more passion, attraction, and sexual satisfaction in our lives. Who doesn't want more of all of that?

There are five different Blueprints Types in this system. There is no hierarchical order to them; there is no one that is "better" than another. We all have the capacity to explore and express each one of them too. Think of all five of them layered as in a five-tiered cake. The predominate or primary Blueprint can be thought of as the largest layer. The other four are there too, in varying degrees of thickness. The height of each layer and the order in which they're stacked in the layer cake plays a role on the road to your turn-on.

With all that said, let's introduce you to the Erotic Blueprints. The first is the *Energetic* Blueprint. People with this as their primary Blueprint are referred to as "Energetics." Energetics like the tease, and they adore the state of longing and anticipation. Delightfully, their turn-on frequently starts long before either partner initiates touch. They get turned on by their partner's turn-on too. Those with this Blueprint often feel like (and are sometimes told) that they are too sensitive to energies. The truth is that they can be extremely sensitive. If this sensitivity is regarded with appropriate care and attention, it can actually be an incredible gift. It's like having highly attuned, extra sensory perception. Such sensitivity has its downside, or shadow, and can cause an Energetic to short-circuit and shut down instantaneously when sexual touch comes too quickly or otherwise isn't timed effectively. A seductive tease, intimate eye contact, breathing techniques, and sacred sexual practices are all fantastic ways to get this Blueprint Type in the mood.

Those with the *Sensual* Blueprint at the forefront naturally have a deep connection to all five senses. They have the capacity for intense body awareness if they can get out of their heads and relax into their body and let it do what it does best: feel sensation. These types like everything to be "just so" in order to engage sexually and are happiest when the mood is set for an intimate encounter. They enjoy arranging the music, lighting, and scents all to their fancy. While repairing the sensual disconnect is an effective tool for all Blueprints, as we discussed in Chapter Three, it's especially true for this Blueprint. When things aren't right in their surroundings, orgasm can be elusive, but when everything is to their liking, they can truly let go of the head chatter and drop into their body. Once relaxed, deep, multisensory orgasms are possible. Pleasurably focusing on any one of their senses is a great start. Sensual massages, hot baths, and candlelit dinners are all high on the list of those with this Blueprint.

The *Sexual* Blueprint is pure and simple; all kinds of direct genital stimulation of a sexual nature is the name of their game. Arousal comes from friction, pressure, nudity, and/or sexual imagery. They want orgasm; otherwise, why bother? Most of us have been enculturated toward accepting this Blueprint as the "right" way to be. Those with this Blueprint as their predominant type are, well, highly sexual and need to engage in sex to feel released, relaxed, or loved. They are easy to please and arouse and make wonderful, fun lovers. Turning them on is simple: get naked, get to it, and get 'em done, *and often*. It's almost foolproof for this Blueprint Type! Without the ability to properly communicate, the *Sexual* Blueprint can create trouble in a partnership. They often get too focused on orgasm without enjoying the ride and have a narrow definition of what *sex* is. A reliance on porn can be especially problematic for this Blueprint Type. With effective methods for communicating their needs and desires, along with learned skills to deeply listen to the needs and desires of the sexual partners they choose, those with a Sexual Blueprint can partner with other types without problem.

Then there are those who are wired for kink. The *Kinky* Blueprint Types derive deep pleasure from everything that they regard as naughty or outside of what they view as "normal." Sometimes, this doesn't even need to involve genital touch, physical arousal, or orgasm, as is the case with psychological kink, where the turn-on happens in their head. For someone turned on by the physical sensations of kink, the very feeling of a rope wrapped around their wrist or waist gets them going. While there is often overlap between having the Kinky Blueprint and the lifestyle or practice of BDSM, this is not always the case. The *Kinky* Blueprint explores what is taboo for them however they choose to define *taboo*. For one person, it literally could mean having sex with the lights on; for another, sex in front of other people; for a third, surrendering to the power of someone who dominates them. People with this Blueprint can be very creative and communicative, but they often have trouble admitting their type because of the culturally imposed shame associated with it. Without a strong understanding of how to engage and play safely with this Blueprint, people with this Blueprint Type can put themselves (or others) in danger. Turning this type on requires pushing their edges, taking them out of their comfort zone, and experimenting with what they consider "forbidden."

The *Shapeshifter* Blueprint is a combination of all of the above Blueprints. People who are true "Shapeshifters" are well-versed in all four Blueprint styles of intimacy and are aroused by all of them. While most of us can occasionally dabble and play with the other Blueprints, a Shapeshifter needs to experience and engage with aspects of all four Blueprint Types on the road to sexual satisfaction. Knowing the vast nature of their turn-on means a Shapeshifter can please and is pleased by any type of lover. Shapeshifters want it all, and they always want more. Partners sometimes struggle to track the Shapeshifter's ever-changing desires and needs. Unaware of their Shapeshifter nature, many with this Blueprint have a tendency to please their partner rather than get their own needs met. A Shapeshifter's work, therefore, is to figure out what they want in any given moment and communicate it effectively. If their partner can then receive that communication, they will find it possible to please the voracious appetite of the Shapeshifter.

Just like with the Quodoushka teachings, we are merely giving you a small taste of the Erotic Blueprints. Both of these systems can work wonders for you in discovering more about your sexual core. Be sure to complete Prescription 10, where you can take a free, online quiz to discover your primary Erotic Blueprint Type and how the other layers of your cake are stacked. Knowing how you reach turn-on can greatly improve your sex life. Try it on for yourself! We have a hunch it will fit you to perfection!

Sexual Expression

As you just learned, there is significant variation in what turns people on. Who we express and share our turn on with varies greatly as well. Relationships come in many configurations. There are also many ways to express yourself sexually.

A *relationship configuration* refers to *how* we love, not *who* we love. In our society, most people follow one type of relationship configuration: one that is monogamous, meaning each person has one long-term partner at a time. There is nothing wrong with this relationship configuration. Yet, when *any* particular relationship structure dominates popular culture, we tend to view it as "normal" and everything else as "abnormal." If you feel that a monogamous relationship is right for you, that's great. However, there are other partnerships that do exist. Some people are in a relationship with more than one person (polyamorous). Some relationships are non-monogamous or open, and some partnerships occasionally add another person to their sex play. The relationship configurations described may be just as healthy as a monogamous one as long as the communication is honest and clear with all partners.

Sexual expression varies far beyond relationship configurations. Some women prefer solo sex, while others prefer a committed partner or a series of partners. Some like quickies, while others like to be devoured in long, luxurious lovemaking sessions lasting for hours. Some express themselves in the privacy of their own home, while others derive great pleasure from being witnessed by a group. There are *so many healthy ways* to enjoy sex and sexuality, and it's not up to us to decide which ones speak to you.

That said, we do stress the importance of exploring the boundaries of your comfort zone. We want you to walk toward the edge without falling off. Why? Well, it's because there is such a thing as a rut, and if you've found yourself less interested in sex for any reason, you may have inadvertently fallen into one. As humans, we tend not to venture too far from what's easy, quick, and familiar. But the truth about turn-on is that it changes day by day, often moment by moment. We're not in the same mood every day; most of us don't like having the exact same type of sex over and over any more than we like eating the same meal day in and day out.

One way to find your way around your comfort zone is to explore the realm of fantasy. And here, like nearly every other aspect of women's sexuality, no two women are alike. Some have active fantasy lives. There are other women who don't fantasize at all. But if you're in a rut, exploring fantasy may provide an opportunity to carve a new pathway out.

There are other ways to get unstuck too. You can start by playing with positions (even in self-pleasuring!), exploring different types of stimulation, and, yes, trying out sex toys—which we'll look at more clearly in Chapter Seven. The following prescriptions may also help you gently push the boundaries of your comfort zone.

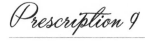

Vulva Selfie

This prescription helps you get to know your vulva on a more intimate level, appreciating it in all its glory.

A note on technology: As most of us know, photos can be tricky to erase these days. If your phone is set to automatically back up your photos, you may want to delete the selfie you take fairly quickly or disable the automatic backup. If you have kids, professional contacts, or anyone else who may have access to your phone, a picture of your gorgeous vulva, while it may impress them with its beauty, may not be appropriate to keep around. In other words: be wise about what happens with this photograph. Use your best judgment.

What You'll Need:

- Fifteen minutes of complete privacy.

- Good lighting.

- Your cell phone.

- Paper.

- Colored art supplies such as markers, paints, or colored pencils.

Let's Get Started!

- Get out your phone and remove your clothing from the waist down.

- Arrange the lighting just-so; you can use the selfie camera, or front camera, to see what you're doing.

- Now, take a selfie of your vulva. Yes, a selfie. Yes, of your vulva. It may take a few shots to get the most accurate representation.

- Using paper and your art supplies, draw the vulva in the picture. Really study the curves, folds, crevices, and creases. Notice the value and variety of its color. Notice the size and the proportions, the length of the hood and the thickness of the tissue, and see how these may relate to the type of pleasure you most enjoy. Have fun with this study!

- It's up to you to decide what to do with this piece of art once you're finished. Cover it in glitter? Sure! Frame it and put it over the mantle? Sing to it, offer it flowers, or bury it ceremonially in the backyard? Totally your call! This beautiful vulva is all yours, and all that we ask is that you treat it with reverence.

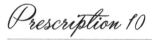
Prescription 10

Find Your Erotic Blueprint

You may already have a sense of which of the five Erotic Blueprint Types you are after having read about them above. There's also a chance you're still wondering. In either case, there's an online quiz you can take that will help you determine your Erotic Blueprint Type. Our hope is that you will take the quiz and discover a pathway to your turn-on that ultimately will help increase your pleasure.

What You'll Need:

- Ten-plus minutes of complete privacy.

- A cell phone, computer, or tablet, possibly using an incognito tab if it is a shared device and you are concerned about privacy.

- An email address where you can receive your results.

Let's Get Started!

- Take the Erotic Blueprint quiz at http://bit.ly/QuizwVL.

- Fill out the answers, put in your email address, and receive your results!

- We hope you dive into Jaiya's work and discover how understanding your Erotic Blueprint can give you access to the most fulfilling types of pleasure for you.

Prescription 11

Write Your Sexiest Story

As we discussed in this chapter, fantasizing is a great way to get yourself out of a rut. Some fantasies are wild and exotic, while others are more like ideas and thoughts of pleasurable things.

For this prescription, we're asking you to write your wildest or mildest story about sex, where you're the main character. Your sexiest story may be full-on erotica, or it may not even involve sex at all. It may include a sexual experience that you're dying to live out in the real world or an idea that turns you on but that you would never act out in your everyday life. This is just for you, and there's no right or wrong way to do it. Remember, that's why it's called *fantasy*! The goal is to help you discover more about who you are at your sexual core.

Get writing and see what surprises you. Perhaps you're more creative than you realize!

What You'll Need:

- Up to thirty minutes of complete privacy.

- A journal and a pen.

- Your imagination and creativity.

Let's Get Started!

- First, set the mood. Light a candle; put some music on; pour yourself a glass of wine, tea or strong coffee—whatever works for you!

- Begin to imagine something that turns you on. Again, it doesn't have to be sexual, necessarily; it only needs to evoke the feelings that make you feel the most sexual.

- Now, start writing! Have fun with it; this is your story. Let it take you wherever it wants to go.

- At the end of this prescription, you can keep or destroy your sexy story. (And, of course, if you liked the prescription, you can always write another one!)

Knowing Yourself on a Whole New Level

These internal aspects we have discussed in this chapter lie at the heart of your sexual core. From your special, beautiful anatomy to your own set of turn-ons to the way you choose to express your sexuality, you've come to know the unique set of characteristics that make you who you are as a sexual being. Understanding this helps you get to know yourself on a whole new level. Just like the external influencers affecting your sexual core are always in flux, your internal aspects are often growing and changing too, albeit more slowly. Mapping your sexual core as a whole is an ongoing process.

It's also a lifelong practice, as Sarah learned through her work with Elizabeth. Sarah became an avid user of both the Erotic Blueprints™ and the teachings of the Quodoushka. From there, she fell in love with her vulva, told her boyfriend how she wanted to be touched, and used the Erotic Blueprints to create a really hot relationship with him. It turned out they were a great match!

But she didn't stop self-pleasuring. In Sarah's case, self-pleasuring was always going to be a big part of her sexual life—an idea that we suggest you consider for yourself. In the next chapter, we'll explore more about making a self-pleasure practice a regular part of your healthy lifestyle. We're going to include deeper penetration as a part of that exploration. Armed with your commitment to learning and understanding the intimate inner workings of your sexual core, you're ready to deepen your practice and find the mind-blowing pleasure that awaits you.

CHAPTER SEVEN

Deepening Your
Self-Pleasure Practice

A Note from Dee:

Danielle came in because sex with her husband hurt. She was married and thirty years old. When they started dating, she was intimidated by the size of his penis; however, for well over a year, they had enjoyed a rich and full sex life where "foreplay seemed to last for days on end."

Then, they got married. Their work and social lives were busy, which left little time for sex. As time when on, "ABC" sex became the norm—which means having sex only on 'A'nniversaries, 'B'irthdays, and 'C'hristmas. As a result, sex started to hurt—a lot. She now winced at the very thought of him entering her. Because of the pain, they had more oral sex, which they both enjoyed; however, over time, they felt it wasn't enough. Danielle missed the foreplay and wanted more pleasurable and frequent penetrative sex.

After talking about her husband and their marriage, I had no reason to believe that their relationship was the problem. Yet I wondered what had caused the shift—if they'd had pain-free sex for a year, why was his size such a problem now?

I first assured Danielle that pain with intercourse was not uncommon and something we could address. Then, I asked her more questions about when sex started to hurt.

Danielle listed several things that happened during that time period, none of which seemed to fully explain the source of her pain. Then, with embarrassment, she told me about something that happened once when having sex before they were married. They'd been having great sex "for hours." She remembers being incredibly turned on as she had an amazing but "weird" orgasm. Afterward, they realized that her orgasm had soaked the sheets. She was horrified, thinking she'd "wet" their bed. After that, she was afraid it would happen again and was way more nervous about having sex.

Danielle was embarrassed about what had happened and still felt some shame. I knew that she had not wet the bed. What had happened was an experience known as female ejaculation. After feeling so horrified, it was understandable that she was nervous about sex. And I suspected that infrequent penetration had, in turn, also negatively affected her pelvic floor muscles, leaving them tighter than they should be. Once the muscles were overly tight, they made penetration more difficult, creating a cycle that was difficult to break. To top it off, her fear of "wetting the bed" again, kept her from fully enjoying partnered sex.

My suspicions about Danielle's pelvic floor muscles were confirmed during my physical examination. As a result, I suggested that using vaginal dilators would be a way to help her reacquaint herself with her vagina and get her pelvic floor muscles working properly again. We talked about the incident of "wetting the bed," and I explained why it was nothing to be ashamed of—a topic we'll cover in detail at the end of this chapter. She laughed, relieved to hear that she wasn't peeing on herself at the ripe ole age of thirty! We also talked about how the dilators would help her pelvic floor muscles relax, her anxiety to ease, and her function to return, allowing for more pleasurable and frequent pen-

etration. It wouldn't be quick or easy; I told Danielle that she would have to work at it for a while, just as she would if she were training any other muscle in her body. But she felt much more confident about herself, and I knew that would help her on her way. Danielle left my office with a clear set of instructions in her hands, a little bag of dilators in her purse, and a smile on her face.

N ow that you've improved your understanding of yourself as a sexual being, it's time for you to step up your self-pleasure practice. Dee sent Danielle home with a set of practices and tools to help her become more comfortable with penetration. At the end of this chapter, we'll offer the same set of prescriptions to you.

We ask that you to spend quite a while integrating this chapter because it covers a lot of ground. Please allow yourself enough time. It requires you to strike a delicate balance between diminishing pain if necessary and expanding into your pleasure. We ask you to be gentle as this process unfolds, returning to the prescriptions we've already given you to support you along the way. It's possible that you'll need to return to this chapter's prescriptions many times before getting to the end of the book.

In this chapter, we'll explain how you can make self-pleasure a practice and why it's so important to do so. If, like Danielle, you experience pain with penetration, we'll discuss how using vaginal dilators can help you understand your limits and how to work gently and safely through them. We'll teach you how to prepare yourself for penetration, eventually arriving at blood-pumping, heart-thumping, hips-humping arousal before putting anything inside your vagina. And then, once your body is at a state of high arousal, we'll explain how to have penetrative sex that feels really good. For those who desire a more advanced personal practice, we've included a section in the prescriptions on how to locate your G-spot.

Let's start with looking at self-pleasure as an ongoing practice.

The Importance of Practice

We've all heard that "practice makes perfect." And while we're not so sure there *is* a perfect when it comes to women's pleasure, we know that practicing certainly makes everything better. If we pick up a new sport, try to play an instrument, or even learn a new card game, we don't expect ourselves to immediately excel at it. We know that we'll have to train our bodies and minds in order to reach higher levels of play. To attain a goal, we need both a *will* and a *way*. Most of this book has been dedicated to providing you with a way to *increased pleasure*. The will piece, however, is up to you. We can encourage you, but we can't make you practice.

Luckily, as recent advancements in neuroscience show us, will can grow over time with proper incentives, like pleasure. It's part of the idea of neuroplasticity that we introduced way back in Chapter Two. When our brains reward us for a behavior by flooding us with dopamine, we associate the behavior as positive and are more likely to repeat it.[56]

That's why engaging in a new behavior frequently, making a pattern out of it, helps us get out of old patterned behavior. The more we receive a reward (which could be physical pleasure or, at the beginning, even telling ourselves what a great job we did), the more likely we are to repeat the pattern. Eventually, performing the behavior becomes automatic, instead of a conscious choice that we have to sit down and think about. In other words, we form a habit.[57]

This starts with conscious choice—by saying to ourselves, "I am going to make self-pleasure a regular practice." As author Martha Beck explains in her book, *The Four-Day Win,*

> The 4-day repetition is necessary to fully install a skill into the hardwiring of your brain. Four daily iterations break through the feeling that you're a novice and make you think of the skill or activity as "something I do." For instance, if you've gone snowboarding, eaten at a certain restaurant, or

played poker on just one occasion, and someone asks you about snowboarding or going to that restaurant or playing cards, you'll think, "Yeah, I tried that once." If you've done the activity twice, you still won't think of yourself as "someone who does that," only as "someone who's done that a *couple of times*." After three experiences, you'll probably think and say, "I've done that a *few* times." If you're like most of the people I've quizzed, it's around the fourth iteration that the activity changes in your mind from "something I did a few times" to "something I do." Yes, I snowboard. Yes, I eat at that restaurant. Yes, I play poker.[58]

So, take a look at what works best for you and your schedule. We recommend that you make a goal for self-pleasuring—once a week at the very least, twice a week is even better, and three times a week means you're really going strong! You obviously have to be realistic about it, but we encourage you to take your practice through the roof whenever and however you can. *Making time for your pleasure is essential, and well worth it.*

While forming a self-pleasuring habit, you may experience some resistance. In fact, this is often part of the process of habit formation. There's a long-standing myth that habit formation takes just twenty-one days, but it has been thoroughly debunked by more recent science, which shows that it can take much longer for a new habit to stick.[59] During that time, you're likely to face any number of challenges: busyness, laziness, pattern disruption (by illness, vacation, etc.), or thoughts like *"this isn't working"* or *"OK, enough already, I've already figured it out."* But to make lasting change, you'll have to push through this resistance and keep going.

If we stop midway when forming a new habit, we typically have to go back to the beginning. On a physical level, our muscles can atrophy; our tissues and cells can forget what they were learning to do. On a psychological level, we have to get ourselves psyched up to start forming the habit again. If you do get bumped back to the beginning, be kind to yourself and start again. It's the only way to make a change. An accountability partner may help. Give one of your sisters or favorite friends this book and suggest you become pleasure practice buddies. Report on your struggles and triumphs. Do whatever it takes to keep yourself motivated and working toward the goal of feeling more pleasure in your body!

Lucky for you, we're helping you build what should turn into a pretty fun habit: self-pleasuring. And the rewards, from the perspective of brain chemistry, are both significant and cumulative. Make time for your pleasure and *it will increase*. That's a promise!

Reassessing Your Pain

For most women who have pain with sex, penetration is the central trigger. Since this chapter involves penetration, it's important for us to go back and check in with any pain you may have had. How is it now? Has it changed?

If, for any reason, you skipped over sections of Chapter Two in this book, please go back and review them now. We believe that anyone addressing chronic pain in any part of their body needs to understand how pain works in a general sense. It's also paramount to know the context around women's sexual pain—namely, how it's treated (or not), what it's called, and how the medical community approaches its healing.

Finally, at the risk of boring you by restating it too many times, we need to say the following for anyone who may have missed it: pain with penetration, be it from a tampon, a finger, a toy, a gynecological exam, or sex itself, is a big deal. It matters. Painful sex is *common*, but that doesn't make it *okay*. If you are still experiencing pain with penetration, be exceedingly gentle with yourself moving forward.

We have you working on your own for a reason. As researchers noted, "Vulvodynia results in significant disruptions to the sexual, relational, and psychological functioning of affected women and their romantic partners, and these consequences can be just as distressing as the pain itself."[60] This is part of why we're taking you through this process on your own, without your partner's direct involvement. Working on your own during this particularly difficult phase of healing may give you the space you need to address your emotions. But you can still include your partner by explaining what's going on. Share what you're doing with your partner and ask for support as you move through the process.

And working through it can have great benefits. Let's take Danielle, whom you met at the beginning of the chapter, as an example. Though we're not big fans of the phrase, "use it or lose it," it works well here. Danielle and her husband hadn't been having much sex; when sex is very infrequent, the mucosal tissue at the opening of the vagina changes, which, for Danielle, caused pain with penetration. Her anxiety and worry about wetting the bed with orgasm caused her pelvic floor muscles to overly tighten, leaving her with little chance of normal function. In unison, this combination of biological and psychological influencers made it harder to accommodate her well-endowed husband. As Danielle made her way through the series of vaginal dilator exercises, her pelvic floor muscle function returned, allowing her to use the largest dilator without pain.

Sounds pretty good, right? We want to help get you there. As you go through these practices, pain may arise. If that happens, it's important to look at its dynamic nature. Most pain doesn't just turn on and stay on at 100 percent of its strength. Instead, there's usually some ebb and flow taking place. Pay attention to this.

Pain Scale

No Pain

0 – Pain free.

Mild Pain
Nagging, annoying but doesn't really interfere with daily activities.

1 – Pain is very mild, barely noticeable. Most of the time you don't think about it.
2 – Minor pain. Annoying and may have occasional stronger twinges.
3 – Pain is noticeable and distracting; however, you can get used to it and adapt.

Moderate Pain
Interferes significantly with daily activities.

4 – Moderate pain. If you were deeply involved in an activity, it can be ignored for a period of time but is still distracting.
5 – Moderately strong pain. It can't be ignored for more than a few minutes, but with effort you still can manage to work or participate in some social activities.
6 – Moderately strong pain that interferes with normal daily activities. Difficulty concentrating.

Severe Pain
Disabling; unable to perform daily activities.

7 – Severe pain that dominates your senses and significantly limits your ability to perform normal daily activities or maintain social relationships. Interferes with sleep.
8 – Intense pain. Physical activity is severely limited. Conversing requires great effort.
9 – Excruciating pain. Unable to converse. Crying out and/or moaning uncontrollably.
10 – Unspeakable pain. Bedridden and possibly delirious. Very few people will ever experience this level of pain.

Remember this?

Using the pain scale provided above, we also want you to rate your pain from 0–10. Throughout this practice, if you feel pain, assess its level. Monitoring your pain may help you gain some sense of control over it as you learn techniques to make it better. Just as you watch your pain go up and down, you can track the progress of your arousal. Ideally, you'll be working toward low levels of pain and high levels of pleasure. Let's take another look at the Pleasure Calibration Scale™:

The Pleasure Calibration Scale™

0 – Ain't nothin' going on here.

1 – Huh. This might be interesting!

2 – Oh! I think I feel something!

3 – Wow! Alrighty then. Let's keep this going!

4 – I'm cooking now! This is amazing!

5 – OMG! Don't stop, don't stop!

And eventually...

6 – Wheeeee! Here I come!

And how about this?

For the sake of simplicity, we'll say that when you start this practice, penetration is *completely off limits* until you reach at least pleasure level 4. As you continue to work with your own pleasure and pain, you may start experimenting with penetration slightly earlier to find your limit. It's our hope that by the time your arousal hits pleasure level 5 or 6, your vulvar pain will have eased. As a matter of fact, Dee prescribes orgasms (pleasure level 6) to her patients after their pain has lessened, as the very best time to attempt penetration is often just following an orgasm. So your goal with this practice is to monitor your pain *and* your pleasure, finding your own optimal moment for penetration. Later, if you choose to share this with a partner, such knowledge will be indispensable.

In Chapter Two, we introduced the idea that the vaginal canal becomes more supple as arousal increases blood flow and decreases tension in the pelvic floor muscles. This was precisely what worked for Danielle; as she learned to release the tension in her pelvic floor muscles, she simultaneously worked to increase her arousal. By doing so, she found that her husband's size was no longer an issue.

A Note from Dee:

With sufficient arousal, the entire landscape of the vulva changes as blood rushes to the tissue, plumping up the area. As engorgement increases, so does sensitivity. The swelling pushes pleasure mechanoreceptors to the surface of the skin where they are more receptive to stimulation. As they are highly sensitive, they can now experience greater pleasure from touch, temperature change, and even simple airflow.

There are other visible changes that accompany engorgement. The clitoris may become more visible in some as it becomes erect, while in others, it seems to retract. The labia majora also swell and draw back, just as the pelvic floor muscles relax, opening the vulva slightly. The labia minora typically become puffy, change color, and produce natural lubrication, though with some there's no visible sign of wetness. The clitoral bulbs running along the insides of the vaginal opening, while not as sensitive as the clitoris itself, can also increase in size, slightly narrowing the vaginal opening. The entire area gets warmer from the increased blood flow, becoming more supple.

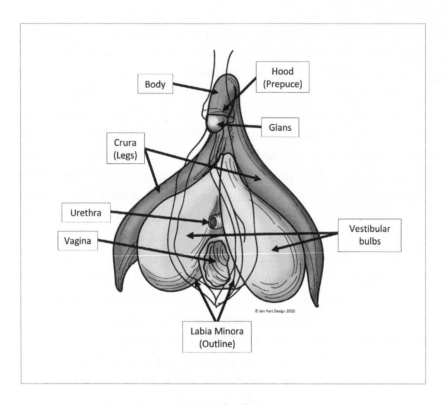

Remember her?

As your arousal increases and decreases on the calibration scale, note how your body is responding. Remember *reflexive splinting*? It could pop up here as the automatic protective response that causes tension throughout the body, including the pelvic floor muscles. The muscles typically clench when anticipating pain with penetration. Breathing deeply helps to calm the entire nervous system. Refer back to the breathing exercises described in Chapter Two. You can learn to retrain the brain and the body by providing a more positive experience.

Throughout the process, continue to remind yourself that *you are the one in control of what is happening*. This can have transformative effects too. When we realize we have a certain measure of control over our body, we reduce fear, thereby reducing tension. We retrain our brains to the positive experience. Touching your vulva and penetrating your vagina in your own time and way is safe, joyful, and positive as you work through pain with pleasure. You've got this. Pleasure *is* possible!

The Occurrence of Female Ejaculation

Danielle noted the amazing but weird orgasm that took place while having sex with her husband after she'd reached an incredible state of turn on, which Dee explained to her was *female ejaculation.* Technically speaking, female ejaculation is characterized as the spontaneous expulsion of fluid that can happen after a specific part of the of the vaginal wall, or the G-spot, is stimulated or after an extended period of clitoral stimulation. It is a clear or milky fluid that flows out of a woman's urethra. The amount of ejaculate released ranges from very little to a whole lot. It's yet another thing that varies from woman to woman.

Now, we need to let you know up front that the science itself is annoyingly unclear on this—there is no clear consensus on what the phenomenon is, exactly what it consists of, or why it happens when it does, and only in some women. We don't know if all women are physically capable of it. There's even some debate as to whether there are multiple types of female ejaculation. All we know for sure—and what we want to pass on to you—is that it *does* happen sometimes for some women, and *it is nothing to be ashamed of!* In fact, there are many people who really enjoy it and create the right situation—aka the right type of stimulation—for female ejaculation to occur on a regular basis. It can be a massive turn-on!

A Note from Elizabeth:

> *Female ejaculation is a magical, mystical, but certainly-not-mythical phenomenon. It's sometimes referred to as* squirting. *Historical accounts of this phenomenon go back over two thousand years and come from around the globe. It*

has been described in Chinese, Roman, Japanese, and Indian cultures—the final of which calls female ejaculate amrita, or the "nectar of the Gods." I know sex educators who can teach the technique but haven't ejaculated themselves; I also know plenty of women who, like Danielle, have ejaculated unexpectedly and thought they peed. Some women have been able to ejaculate with certain partners but not with others, or only at certain points of their lives. Some women think it feels incredible and some don't, while others barely take notice that it happens.

Many women note that just before they ejaculate, it feels like they have to pee. If you feel this sensation while being penetrated and you know your bladder is empty, it may be a worthwhile experiment to just roll with the sensation and see what happens. For some women, it just flows, while for others, they follow the urge to bear down like they're pushing out a tampon, and this is what causes them to ejaculate.

The main take-home here is that the only norm, when it comes to female ejaculation, is variation. If it happens, it's normal. If it doesn't, it's normal too. Relax and have fun either way![61]

As you begin to penetrate your vagina, you have a greater chance of locating and stimulating your G-spot. If you are able to locate and then choose to stimulate your G-spot, ejaculation may or may not happen. Most women require extended G-spot stimulation to ejaculate; however, others can ejaculate after achieving high levels of arousal from external stimulation of the entire vulva. The experience of female ejaculation is not the same sensation as clitoral orgasm. The two experiences are different, although one can accompany the other.

If you experienced female ejaculation and were self-conscious about it, but are curious to try again, you can protect the bed by putting a towel down before self-pleasuring or having sex. A lot of women who ejaculate on a regular basis have mattress protectors or use what are known as "splash pads" to eliminate the worry of wetting or ruining their mattresses. These are suggested items to use as you experiment with your body and explore female ejaculation for yourself.

Preparing for Deep Penetration

By now, you should understand that pain often decreases with arousal. Because of this, it's important for you to get yourself fully aroused before you even dream of putting anything in your vagina! Use Prescriptions 1–11 to help you prepare. Relax your muscles, admire your beautiful vulva in the mirror, connect with your sensuality, and touch your body softly. Lubricate, lubricate, lubricate, and stimulate your clitoris. All of these are uncompromisable prerequisites to penetration! And if you can, have an orgasm. It will make penetration easier.

To experiment with penetrative pleasure, starting with your fingers is always best; with skin-to-skin contact, you'll be able to feel the differences in temperature, in varying textures, and will be able to identify any tension that may be present inside your vagina. But eventually, the prescriptions will ask you to work your way up to using a sex toy specifically designed for penetration.

There are many toys out there for you to choose from. And these days, most sex shops sell them online and deliver them in discreet packaging. Many US cities and even some progressive rural areas have sex shops that cater to women, often with women on staff to help you through all that's available so you make the right purchase for your need. These employees and business owners are used to first-time customers who feel a little nervous, so if that's you, don't be shy; get in there!

Some toys vibrate; others don't. Those that vibrate either use batteries or are rechargeable. Toys are commonly made from plastic or silicon, but you may prefer surgical grade steel or glass, which can be warmed or chilled prior to use. For the purposes of these prescriptions, it doesn't much matter. Toys can be straight, ridged, or curved. Some are flexible, while some are rigid. Those designed specifically to reach the G-spot are curved to stimulate the front wall of the vagina. Toys can come with all sorts of bells and whistles; while we haven't seen it yet, we're sure someone is hard at work inventing a whistling toy somewhere! But for the purpose of these prescriptions, the simpler the better.

For those of you who have a history of pain when anything was inserted into your vagina, you'll need a set of *vaginal dilators* to address that pain. Dilators look a lot like toys but are actually tools designed for expanding the vaginal opening. They come in a graded set that gets progressively larger. Some sets are firm, while others are soft. We recommend that you purchase a full, graduated set so you can increase your tolerance slowly.

The prescriptions that follow are advanced, and it's up to you to know your limits when using them. That said, if you've followed along with the prescriptions throughout the book, you have all the tools you need to go forward. We suggest that you make sure you are truly ready for deep penetration before attempting it. In other words, if you read through this chapter and decide you aren't ready, just keep practicing Prescriptions 1–11 until you are.

You'll know you're ready when you're thoroughly familiar with how to stimulate your vulva to the point of full engorgement. You've felt arousal course through your body and are excited, perhaps even aching, to try penetrating your vagina—even if you still feel protective, which is normal and healthy. This is the level of desire that indicates your body is ready for penetration; any arousal state less than this means penetration is premature.

Prescription 12

Using Vaginal Dilators

If the thought of using dilators makes you want to scream and run away, please read on before skipping this prescription! We are *not* going to ask you to progressively insert larger and larger dilators into your vagina and keep them there for ten to twenty minutes while you writhe in pain.

We prefer a more functional approach, helping you to teach your body how it should respond to penetration. The goal of the prescription is for you to progress from the smallest to the largest dilator that you can insert and remove, contract and relax around, with no discomfort. This may not be the largest in your dilator set, but we don't want you to stop at the smallest one either. It's about increasing your ability to accommodate penetration without your body stopping you. For this prescription, you'll need a graduated set of vaginal dilators. Do your research; dilators vary. Check online to find a set that could work for you. What we're focusing on in this prescription is tracking, breathing through, and ultimately reducing pain, with and during penetration. With the dilators, you'll be using your pelvic floor muscles along the way to help rewire your brain's response to any pain that occurs.

Just a reminder—we're not suggesting that the pain is all in your head. Reflexive splinting is a huge problem; when there's pain produced at the vulva or in the vagina, the pelvic floor muscles come to the rescue by attempting to "close the door" to the opening, keeping anything from penetrating further. That response not only decreases the size of the vaginal opening, it also creates pain and burning at the vulva. The physical struggle is quite real but one that you can change using progressively sized insertable dilators and active pelvic floor muscle actions.

The exercise is simple: you'll insert a dilator, actively contract and relax your pelvic floor muscles around it, and then remove it. Finding the right dilator can be tricky, though. If the dilator is too comfortable (pain level 0), it's too small. We're looking for mild (pain level 1 or 2) pain—the type that you might just describe as "mild" or "annoying." Moderate pain (pain levels 3–6) is too much, and severe pain (pain levels 7–10) should be avoided at all costs. If you cannot insert even the smallest dilator without experiencing moderate pain, keep practicing Prescriptions 2–5, found in Chapter Two. On the other hand, if you are able to insert and remove the smallest one after contracting and relaxing your muscles around it without discomfort, you'll need to begin with the next larger size in your set.

These are the steps that you will take as you progress. Be aware that you will be looking for some discomfort as you progress to a larger-sized dilator. When you get to the point where you experience mild pain (pain levels 1–2) only when you squeeze around the dilator and no pain (pain level 0) when you let go, that's when the brain retraining begins. You learn to override the actions of reflexive splinting (muscle contracting and causing pain) with the knowledge that relaxing the muscles doesn't hurt.

Eventually, you'll return to Prescriptions 2–5 (found in Chapter Two), performing them nightly with your dilator in place.

What You'll Need:

- Fifteen to thirty minutes of uninterrupted privacy at bedtime.

- A set of vaginal dilators.

- Lube. We suggest you follow the dilator manufacturer's recommendations, as there are lubes that work best with specific materials. Don't use silicon lube with silicon toys; it will degrade the material. This is *essential*: please, please lubricate your dilators, and lubricate them well!

- Optional: Extra pillows to prop yourself up.

- Optional: A towel to protect the area below your naked bottom.

- Optional: A journal and a pen.

Let's Get Started!

- Begin by inserting the smallest, well-lubed dilator that causes only mild pain (levels 1 or 2) as described above.

- Then, contract your pelvic floor muscles around the dilator and hold the squeeze for a count of five. Remember that mild pain is *expected* as part of this prescription.

- Maintain your deep breathing pattern that you learned in Chapter Two.

- Let go of the squeeze, feeling your muscles relax.

- Pay attention to when and how your pain increases and decreases. It may be present during both squeeze and release at first. As you make progress, you will find yourself at pain level 0 with your muscles relaxed and pain level 1 or 2 when you squeeze. With continued work, that pain will disappear.

- Continue the pattern of contracting and relaxing for five minutes with the dilator in place.

- Once the five minutes are over, remove the dilator and clean it with a gentle hand soap.

- Congratulations! You've now identified the dilator that's a good fit for you to begin using with Prescription 4 (pelvic muscle exercises).

- Practice Prescriptions 2–5 nightly with your dialtor in place only during the pelvic floor exercises (Prescription 4). Once you are able to complete them with pain level 0, go up to the next size dilator and start again. When you consistently reach pain level 0 with the largest dilator, you can stop performing the prescription.

You may find that you're comfortable moving on to Prescription 13 as you make progress with the dilators. Go for it! Just go slow. Finding pleasure can work wonders on your vulva as well as your brain!

Prescription 13

Experimenting with Deep Penetration

If you're a woman without pain or one who now has pain under control, continue on to this prescription. For those with pain, have a read, but wait until you're fully comfortable with the idea of vaginal penetration.

Please know that we completely understand if you're feeling scared or intimidated by this prescription. Our best advice is to take it slow. You may be able to complete the entire prescription in one go, or it may take you several attempts. *Reach for pleasure* at every turn. Create an environment that pleases your senses—one that's warm, comfortable, and cozy.

Make sure that you're tending to your arousal throughout the process, pausing to stroke your vulva (or using one hand to attend to your clitoris *while* you penetrate yourself with the other), run your hands over your skin, or whatever else might help you stay aroused.

At some point in this process, your hips may begin to move. Let them. They may rock forward and backward or your back may arch just slightly. Your legs may want to move too. Move along with your body's own natural rhythm; listen to what it is telling you.

You may also want to make noise. Making sounds can increase

your pleasure! Play with moaning and groaning, perhaps even growling. Give yourself permission to do whatever sounds right.

Remember, you can take this exercise all at once or in steps. It's really up to you! The point is that it's a *positive* and *desired* experience. This will help your brain record it as something good. Over time, you'll rewrite the script about penetration—from painful to pleasurable.

What You'll Need:

- Thirty to sixty minutes of uninterrupted privacy.

- After reaching a high state of arousal, you'll need an insertable sex toy or device. Be sure to clean it fully prior to and after use, following the manufacturer's instructions.

- Lube. We suggest natural oils if you'd like—coconut, olive, or almond oil. Or, water-based lube works well too. Since you'll lube with both your fingers and your toy, be sure to check the toy manufacturer's instructions to make sure the two are compatible; some materials don't play well with certain types of lube, so do your homework.

- Optional: Extra pillows to prop yourself up.

- Optional: A mirror and good lighting.

- Optional: A towel to put underneath you or for added protection, a waterproof mattress cover or "splash pad."

- Optional: A journal and a pen.

Let's Get Started!

- Start by making sure the space is sensually pleasing to you.

- By now, you also likely have a sense of how to prepare for self-pleasure. Undress from the waist down (though, again, we'll plug the importance of socks!). Lay the towel down, if you prefer to use one, and situate yourself comfortably over it, propping yourself up with pillows with your knees bent and your thighs spread. Place your hand over your vulva and breathe.

- When you feel ready, apply lube to your fingers and begin to stimulate your entire vulva, including your clitoris in whatever manner you want. You can use any technique you have found arousing. Take your time to reach full arousal, feeling around the opening to your vagina every few minutes.

- If you are able to bring yourself to orgasm, feel free to do so! Don't worry if you aren't, though. The goal here is a fully plumped, aroused vulva—not just the clitoris but the whole thing. Before moving forward, you want to feel tingling, warmth, pulsating, or swelling of your vulva. Take all the time you need to get there.

- Once you're fully aroused, squeeze and release your pelvic floor muscles a few times to tap into their power.

- Begin to move a finger or two up and down your vulva, from your clitoris to the vaginal opening. Reapply lube as necessary.

- When you're ready, pause with your finger at the opening. Just let it rest there for a few moments; experiencing this feeling in stillness and enjoy the subtle sensations.

- Then, slowly insert a finger into your vagina.

- Begin to move your finger around slowly, feeling with the pad, not the fingertip. Be gentle with yourself. No poking, prodding, or fast moving in-and-out motions here. These movements may be new for you, and that's okay. We're asking you to learn something new. The goal is to replace old habits or techniques with ones that offer you more pleasure.

- Feel toward the front wall of the vagina, just an inch or two in, and apply and release light pressure. If you move your finger in and out just a bit, you may notice there is an area of tissue that feels different from the tissue around it, either a bit spongy or like a small bulge. This is the area of the G-spot. If it feels good to apply light pressure there, do so; if not, just note what you feel and move on.

- If and when you're called to do so, insert a second finger, and if it feels good, even a third. Begin to slowly glide them in and out, following your body's natural rhythm.

- As your arousal increases, periodically turn your fingers toward the front wall of your vagina again and see if the area feels any different due to the arousal. It may feel like a grape under the skin. If and when it swells, stimulate it directly by pulling against it as you draw your fingers partially out of your vagina. If this feels really, really good, keep doing it! If it doesn't, simply return to pleasurable sensations.

- Once you're familiar with your vagina and have used your fingers to identify what feels really good, it's time, if you'd like, to get out a sex toy and continue to explore pleasure.

- Don't forget to use your lube both around the vaginal opening and on the toy. Hold it against your vaginal opening with one hand while stimulating your entire vulva or just the clitoris with the other.

- When you've reached yet another state of high arousal, slowly ease the toy into your vagina to whatever depth feels good. Don't forget to keep your clitoris happy! Hint: Exhale with your mouth opened wide as you begin to insert the toy. The reason? All circular muscles tend to relax and tighten together; therefore, as you relax your mouth, your pelvic floor muscles follow suit, increasing the size of the vaginal opening.

- Using the toy, explore your vagina. Move it around in different ways and see what new sensations feel good.

- When you feel complete, slowly pull the toy out and relax by placing a cupped hand over your vulva.

- Breathe deeply and be present. Celebrate your success in whatever way works for you.

- Give yourself some time to integrate what just happened, writing in your journal or just lying there, savoring the experience. You did great work today!

- Repeat this prescription often; it never expires.

Your New Lease on Life

We're not going to beat around the bush. This chapter was huge. Just like Danielle was able to do with Dee's help, you learned how to enjoy penetration—or, at least, you began to move in that direction. We looked at why and how practice makes perfect, and how you can continue that practice in a healthy way, being respectful of any pain that arises. We prepared you for deep penetration—something that you probably didn't think was possible when you pulled this book off the shelf—and then, amazingly, you were brave enough to try it. And if you followed our instructions, you're now using the prescriptions again and again. Congratulations! That's no small thing, and we're proud of you!

This concludes Part II of the book. We hope that by now, your relationship with your body and your pleasure have undergone massive transformation! If things went according to plan, you've gotten to know yourself on a whole new level. You've come to understand your pleasure more deeply. You've felt things, physically and emotionally, that you never felt before. You are a whole new woman! And hopefully, you feel a whole lot less pain than you used to, and, as a result, are experiencing more pleasure.

It's likely that others have started to notice. "Have you cut your hair?" they'll ask, or they'll compliment you on your weight. And perhaps you do have a new "do," perhaps you have come closer to a weight that feels good to you (whether it's gaining weight or losing it)—perhaps you're experimenting with changing your outer look to match your new inner experience. In any case, you probably have a renewed lease on life. You have a kick in your step, an energy you never knew was possible. We hope so, at least—it's what we've seen for so many of our clients and patients, and it's what we hope for you. Because the truth is, this is a natural consequence of pleasure! As turn-on increases, self-esteem increases, bringing joy and enthusiasm along with it. And it's nearly always noticeable from the outside.

Up to this point, you've been working on your own. Parts I and II of this book have given you what you need to change your relationship to your sexuality for the better. Part III is for those of you who are in a relationship. Here is where you'll introduce the new, evolved, embodied *you* to your partner. Together as a team, you'll work through the new ideas we present. Get ready, because there's a lot more pleasure coming your way!

If you're looking for a partner, please read these final chapters, as they will help lay a foundation for making your next relationship stronger, more intimate and honest. If you decide to end your journey with us here, put this book down knowing "You're braver than you believe, stronger than you seem, and smarter than you think."[62]

Part Three

The Partnered
Practices

Strategies for Becoming a Better Communicator

Good communication involves both of you listening to what the other has to say, speaking clearly and with intention about your own feelings, using constructive language, and seeking to understand each other's feelings.

Listening is about respect; *be conscious of maintaining and demonstrating respect* throughout this process. It also includes empathy. It's not about agreeing with your partner's feelings; it's about understanding them.

As you listen, focus *on truly understanding what your partner is saying*—don't create a response in your head while the other is talking, and don't get defensive or distracted. This is a huge part of *active listening*, a technique that involves really paying attention to what the speaker is trying to say, regardless of your own viewpoint, and then repeating back what you heard to make sure you understood it correctly. Active listening requires your total focus, care, and comprehension. As you listen to your partner, notice what's really being said. If you didn't understand their words, ask them to please clarify. If you didn't hear them, ask them to repeat. If you want them to be more succinct, ask them to summarize. Lastly, if your advice hasn't been requested, don't offer any.

A Note from Dee:

Everything I learned about communicating, I learned from Glenna.

I met Glenna when I was sixteen. Glenna's husband died suddenly when their six kids were between the ages of three and twelve, leaving her to raise them alone. My boyfriend (now husband) was the youngest. Glenna was a tough woman—she had to be! But she was also extremely nurturing. One of her many wonderful traits was being a fantastic communicator.

She cared about everyone. No matter who you were, she wanted the best for you. She was interested in everything anyone had to say, knowing it was important to them. Glenna didn't reserve her caring or her interest for the people she necessarily agreed with or liked. She took time to listen whenever anyone had something to say. She had a keen way of knowing when people were simply asking, "just hear me." When asked for advice, she gave it with heartfelt care and support.

As my husband and I traverse marriage, parenthood, and now this new journey as grandparents together, we've used Glenna's communication skills throughout our daily interactions, remembering to care about others and demonstrate our genuine interest in their viewpoints. It's pretty simple, actually: just care, be interested, and show it.

A widely known practice that boosts communication skills is the use of *"I" language,* a way of more clearly expressing ourselves. When using "I" language, we take responsibility for what we are thinking and feeling rather than blaming our partners for the way we feel. Instead of saying, "You're always late. You don't care about me," change the wording. "I get really anxious when you don't tell me you're running late" is a more compassionate and less hostile way to communicate your feelings to your partner. It's a more honest way of sharing what's really going on. Over time, practicing this improves our communication.

Another important guideline to follow is to consciously intersperse positive comments to offset the negative ones. *We like the 5:1 rule: five positive comments for every negative one.* Keep the compliments coming! Maintaining a steady flow of positivity will help reduce the sting when you say something negative when angry or feeling hurt.

This may seem obvious but don't take it for granted: if you love your partner, tell them. If you need to apologize, say "I'm sorry."

Don't be afraid to say, "I was wrong," as it's quite powerful. *To be truly received, remember all these things need to be said with sincerity.*

Be careful to *time these conversations appropriately*; don't discuss relationship issues when in bed, whether it's before, during, or after sex. Sure, during sex, you can say, "more of that!" or "a little to the left, please!" but bigger conversations are best left outside the bedroom. Keep the conversations you have in bed positive and short, and stick to subjects that pertain to what's happening in the present moment, answering the question, "What would make this experience even more pleasurable?"

It is also important to *carve out the time you need to have these conversations.* Don't rush into them nor stop them abruptly. Consider splitting the conversation into multiple, bite-size chunks to allow both of you time to integrate what you've talked about.

The more you have these conversations, the less likely things are to pile up. If you've ever known a marriage to break up over an argument about taking out the trash or doing the laundry, you know what we mean. When you spend so much time on the small squabbles, it's nearly impossible to get at what's really going on in your relationship.

And finally, *be sure to do things together that you both enjoy.* The more you enjoy spending time together, the better your communication will be. This is because communication benefits from true intimacy—and, in turn, successful communication helps that intimacy to grow.

There are many clues that might suggest you need to improve the way you communicate. If you find yourself discussing the same issue over and over again without reaching an agreement; if your conversations frequently escalate into arguments; if certain topics are so tense that they're completely off-limits; or if daily communication generally doesn't dip any deeper than small talk, you can be sure that your communication skills deserve an upgrade. The ideas we've provided here can help most people communicate better. If you find yourself truly struggling, it may be necessary to bring in a third party, like a counselor or therapist, to move into the prescriptions in this chapter. Once you're able to communicate openly, your sexual intimacy will immediately benefit.

How Good Communication Builds Sexual Intimacy

In their book, *Undefended Love*, authors Jett Psaris and Marlena S. Lyons define *intimacy* as "direct, unmediated, heart-to-heart connections with ourselves and with others." We love this definition; it describes exactly what a fulfilling romantic and sexual relationship can build. The authors go on:

> Intimacy…can only occur when the heart is *undefended*. To cut through our personal differences, to reach the unveiled part of ourselves that is deep enough to express the most profound and untamed aspects of our being means learning how to love and be loved without defenses and without obstructions. It means cultivating the capacity to be emotionally present even when we feel exposed or vulnerable; learning to relinquish the many strategies we have employed to feel safe and in control; and finding the courage to love without guarantees or requirements. Through developing the capacity for intimacy in this way, we discover love as an abiding presence in the emotional center of our being, our heart, and we can never again feel emotionally disconnected, incomplete, or unloved.[63]

As Psaris and Lyons define it, intimacy is about heart-to-heart connections with others, which is the key ingredient in achieving sexual intimacy. That connection requires strong communication where each partner can comfortably express themselves long before sex even starts. The partners trust that they'll be heard, they know it's safe to ask for what they want, and they're secure enough to negotiate for something different without the other being offended.

A Note from Elizabeth:

By nature, everyone is wired differently. By "everyone" I mean men too. That said, I've noticed a trend when working with couples. Sharing what I've seen may help you understand your partner's way of connecting a little bit better. I want to be really careful here; please understand that what I'll describe is a general trend and not a rule. This won't be a simple Mars versus Venus explanation, either, as we're all way too complicated for that.

Throughout this book, I hope you've learned that many women need to feel connected on an emotional level before they feel safe to express themselves on a sexual level. We've written a lot about it: how to take care of your emotional needs, listen to yourself, and tune in to your inner desires before asking the rest of your body to join the party. These skills helped you become more vulnerable, making the feeling of pleasure all the better. Using the following prescriptions, we hope that you will be able to help your partner tune in as well so that they can access some of those same vulnerabilities and feel more pleasure.

Here's where it gets interesting though. It's easy to assume that tapping into your emotional vulnerability before things get sexual is important for everyone. The truth is not all men, or women for that matter, actually need or want that vulnerability. In fact, talking about his feelings could be as scary for him as talking about having sex may have been for you.

But what if a key to activating a woman's intimate energy is through her emotions, while a key to activating a man's energy is through physical contact? Try this on for size. As a way of connecting, offer some type of physical contact by asking him how he would like to be touched. If what he wants isn't sexual but something like, "Please put your hands on my shoulders for a minute," go for it! Physical contact often helps men access the same intimate energy, vulnerability, and feeling of connection that many women access through their emotional openness. Don't forget that I see this as a trend, not a universal truth. There's a ton of diversity for both men and women in how they feel connected, which might be worth exploring for both of you.

Be curious. Find out what helps him feel safe, secure, and connected to you. For some men it's sex, but for others it's any physical touch. In any case, don't expect that the things that help you feel connected are the same things that help him. Listen, pay attention, and be patient; you might be surprised by what you find!

Now that you've learned about communication and its interplay with intimacy, it's time to break the ice. In the next section, we'll look at ways to do that.

Starting a Conversation about Sex

Having made it this far along in the book, some of you may have already found your way into a conversation about sex. Perhaps you and your partner were able to fall into a comfortable, intimate conversation about sex without even trying. It could be that a natural segue appeared on its own. Perhaps he noticed something different about you. He may have asked you if you'd lost weight or changed your hair, or he may have commented on your extra energy. Over the course of the book, you might have been more open and intimate with him, which increased his level of perceived safety and made him more open and intimate with you. If so, talking about sex probably wasn't that difficult.

Yet there are many of you for whom a conversation about sex simply *hasn't* come up naturally. Throughout your relationship, you never talked about sex, or at least not in a way that felt comfortable to you. If this is your situation, don't wait for the topic to come up; instead, take the plunge by scheduling a good time to talk that works for both of you. No matter how the conversation starts, you're going to have to express yourself and actively listen. You've learned so much about pleasure and pain, and hopefully, you now feel empowered to talk about them with your partner.

As the two of you have this conversation—or, more likely, this series of conversations—watch out for any sign that he's having a hard time. His body may be clearly communicating things he is not able to express verbally, so good listening involves paying close attention. Check for glazed eyes or slumping posture. Notice if he seems stunned, surprised, frustrated, or distracted. Check his hands; is he reaching for his phone, a snack, a beer? Make sure he is engaged and interested. You know this man better than anyone else; you certainly should be able to know whether he's present and able to stay focused on what you have to say.

The first conversation might serve as an icebreaker, easing him into the longer conversation you want to have. Give him a head's up so that he knows what's coming. That way, he may be able to more fully participate. It's possible that he may need some time before really engaging in this type of conversation. Feel free to put the conversation down for a bit—as long as you pick it up again later at an agreed upon time.

This may be the first time he's learning about what's been going on for you—that you were in pain, for instance, or that you weren't having orgasms, if that was your case. Hearing it all at once can be tough on both his heart and his pride. And if you haven't been having sex, it might be a lot for him when you share that you've been self-pleasuring. If he becomes a bit reactive, experiment with resisting the urge to defend yourself. Be sure to frame everything about you. Use "I" language to express yourself: "I didn't know what I needed or wanted, and I couldn't express it to you," or "I needed to understand more about myself. I had no idea how my body worked." It takes great courage to reveal such vulnerability; stay with it, and ask him to remain open to hearing it too.

When you're able to have these sorts of conversations about sex, you'll find there's more room for loving everyday gestures in the relationship.

24/7 Foreplay and Sexy Surprises

Foreplay, in the realm of sex, is a series of actions that aids the process of arousal.

Merriam-Webster's defines *foreplay* as:

1. Erotic stimulation preceding sexual intercourse

2. Action or behavior that precedes an event[64]

We love the second definition because it defines *foreplay* as actions and behaviors. Dee and her husband created the idea of *24/7 foreplay*, which is acting and behaving lovingly and with kindness throughout your relationships twenty-four hours a day, seven days a week.

Both partners have equal responsibility when it comes to fueling sexual desire and arousal. We suggest that you meet that responsibility by looking at your interactions with your partner as a type of foreplay that goes on *all the time*—in other words, 24/7. These acts rarely have anything to do with being sexual; rather, they have everything to do with connecting to and pleasing each other. It's about integrating their happiness in your actions. Implementing 24/7 foreplay can begin with activities such as making the morning coffee, emptying the dishwasher when it's clean, or checking in on your partner's parents without being asked. It's not about keeping score; it's about being mindful. You can never do too many nice things for each other. Consider 24/7 foreplay as daily care and maintenance for your relationship.

One way to enhance 24/7 foreplay is to create sexy surprises. A *sexy surprise* is any unexpected, thoughtful, caring, loving and/

or sexy action you perform for your partner. It's doing something particularly wonderful that they will enjoy. It lets your partner know you are thinking of them, caring for them, or taking care of something on their behalf without being asked.

Some sexy surprises can be pretty sexy. They might involve fulfilling a specific fantasy or offering a sexual experience unexpectedly. Initiating sex can certainly be a sexy surprise for some, especially if you're not the one who usually does so.

But other surprises aren't explicitly sexy; they're measures of sweet kindnesses, instead. Elizabeth once worked with a couple who had two enormous Irish wolfhounds. Actually, *she* had two enormous Irish wolfhounds; *he* generally left all their care to her and wouldn't even let them in his car. Before she arrived home from a business trip, his sexy surprise was to take the dogs for grooming. As she pulled into their driveway, he walked the clean and fresh-smelling dogs out to greet her, complete with bows in their hair. It was a big hit!

The most important rule for a sexy surprise is that you not expect anything in return. The whole purpose of sexy surprises is to practice getting pleasure from giving pleasure; you may get a warm, loving reaction, but the true reward is in giving. It's even better if you can really enjoy the process of planning and executing your sexy surprise. This brings lightheartedness and fun into any relationship.

Integrating 24/7 foreplay and sexy surprises is a wonderful way to increase intimacy between partners, which in turn increases the level of perceived emotional safety each partner feels. It can also increase arousal and turn-on, inviting more sexual contact into the partnership. Twenty-four-seven foreplay, peppered with sexy surprises along the way, becomes a fun game for both partners to play together over time. It forms a strong foundation for healthy, open communication about desires, needs, and both sexual and emotional well-being.

Before giving you the prescription for 24/7 foreplay and sexy surprises, we'll first help you begin an open conversation about sex.

Prescription 14

Having a Conversation about Sex

Though this prescription is presented all at once, it's likely that you'll end up doing it in smaller steps. Getting to the final step of this prescription may take time. We hope this is just the beginning of a greater, ongoing open communication about the sex and sexuality that you and your partner will share.

What You'll Need:

- Twenty-plus minutes of complete, partnered privacy, free of all distractions.

- A timer.

- Comfortable seating for both of you (preferably not on your bed, and certainly not *in* your bed!).

- Space and flexibility to pause and resume conversation as needed.

Let's Get Started!

- Get his agreement to have a conversation with the following guidelines in place.

- As each one of you speaks, be gentle, be kind, and use "I" statements to avoid placing any blame on the other.

- Set the timer for the time you've agreed to. Stick to your upper limit, although the conversation may end before the time is up.

- Begin by telling him what you've been doing and what you've learned from this book. Offer a few specific examples of things that have improved. For instance, you might say, "I didn't know how to have an orgasm and now I do"; "I always hated how my vulva looked and now I think it's beautiful"; or "Before using the prescriptions in the book, I couldn't insert anything into my vagina without feeling pain. Now I can easily use a tampon."

- Tell him what you've learned about your turn-on. Open up about your turn-on and how you're feeding it in different ways.

- Break down your wants, needs, and desires around sex and your partnership. Tell him the ways he turns you on currently, and then offer other ways he may not have considered.

- Then, if he's up for it, invite him to share what he desires. What would turn him on? What would excite him? What does he want from sex and out of your sex life? By asking these questions, you indicate your willingness to hear something that might be difficult for you. Be ready to accept what comes; it's his turn, so don't interrupt.

- Whenever the conversation finishes, be sure to close it intentionally. Make sure both parties are ready to be done for now, and then consider offering physical touch— even if it's a hug. Consider lingering there to soak in the precious moments.

- If things go very well and it moves to more intimate touch or even sex, fantastic! Just make sure the conversation is really closed before you go there.

Prescription 15

24/7 Foreplay and Sexy Surprises

As you've learned, foreplay should happen every day between you and your partner, with sexy surprises sprinkled in along the way. Ideally, you'll begin a fun back-and-forth, but remember that the whole point is to *give* sexy surprises, not to expect anything in return. Implementing 24/7 foreplay and planning your sexy surprises should feel fun and exciting!

What You'll Need:

- We have no idea! It all depends on you and how well you know your partner.

Let's Get Started!

- Start implementing 24/7 foreplay by simply paying attention to your partner and what makes them happy. It has everything to do with connecting to and pleasing the other person. It's about taking care of the small stuff. The most important thing is that you show your partner that you're thinking of them and that you care.

- Then, design a sexy surprise. Go for a grand gesture, something that goes beyond day-to-day maintenance. Do something for them that they haven't done for themselves. Remember, it can be explicitly sexy or not. It doesn't have to cost anything because your action is the gift. Put time and energy into it. Make sure it's meaningful, and make sure it's a surprise!

- When you're ready, implement your surprise! Give it with an open heart, expecting nothing in return. Notice how it feels to please your partner this way.

Upleveling Your Relationship

Most women who work with these communication techniques for a while find that a fulfilling relationship unfolds. The good parts get better, and the challenging parts become less difficult to navigate. As she worked through the prescriptions with her boyfriend, Amanda found that they were able to create a healthy, ongoing conversation about sex and sexuality together.

Our work starts with ourselves. It requires us to look at how we communicate and, especially, how well we listen. When we use communication to build intimacy, it prepares us to have comfortable, open conversations about sex with our partner. We bolster this over time with 24/7 foreplay, looking at sex as the culmination of the love and affection we express throughout our daily lives with our partners.

When you're able to do all of the above, your relationship will make it to the next level, one based on strong, healthy communication. That communicative pattern extends not only to your sex life but to the relationship as a whole.

And with the emotional safety this type of communication provides, you can find the space you need to get really clear on what is welcome and unwelcome at any given moment. Once you and your partner can express whatever is coming up for you in your relationship, you'll have the tools to dive into the intricacies of consent and touch. Read on to find out how you can use your new communication skills to go even deeper as a couple.

CHAPTER NINE

Creating Consent in Your Relationship

A Note from Elizabeth:

Leigh first came into my office nearly a year after her divorce. During the last year of her marriage, and up until the time we met, she'd been in group therapy doing deep work. Her ex-husband had never been supportive; he often mistreated her emotionally and, on occasion, liked rough sex. She never wanted it that way, but endured it, not knowing how to say no.

The couple fell in love and lost their virginity to each other while they were still in high school. They married quite young and had two children shortly thereafter. Their sexual relationship brought Leigh very little pleasure. She told me she never really knew what to do during sex and just let him do whatever he wanted. Leigh never asked for anything different, and her ex-husband didn't seem to care. "I thought that was how sex was supposed to be," she explained. For instance, even though Leigh experienced pain with vaginal intercourse for almost a year after the birth of their second child, she wasn't able to tell her husband about it.

Now in her early forties, Leigh had started dating again. Just before our appointment, Leigh had gone out on several fantastic dates with a childhood friend. The chemistry was there; they both felt an immediate emotional connection. "It's probably too soon to know for sure," Leigh confessed, "but there's definitely a big part of me that hopes this turns into something special. But this time, I want to do things differently. That's why I'm here seeing you."

Leigh wanted a say in what happened in her sex life. She wanted to learn how to say no to things she didn't want, to ask for what she did want, and, most importantly, to be asked before anyone touched her. I really believed that Leigh would benefit greatly if I taught her how to use consent.

In working with me, she discovered a whole lot about her own needs and how to get them met. She also learned to clearly name what she didn't want and say "no" to those things. If her new beau was game, Leigh had the chance to build a relationship rooted in the principles of consent.

The last chapter brought you through the basics of communication with your partner. You now have a stronger skill set when it comes to both listening actively and expressing yourself clearly. Both will come in handy as we explore the ins and outs of giving and receiving consent.

This chapter offers you a conceptual description of consent as well as a way to experience it. It's a huge topic that can be applied to any number of day-to-day circumstances. Take your time reading through this chapter; you may need to go over it several times. It's super important to first understand it intellectually. Once you've got it, we'll then help you explore how consent works with partnered touch and teach you to how to use it effectively in your relationship.

So what is consent, exactly? Well, there are many ways to explain it. Planned Parenthood teaches consent between people using the acronym FRIES, meaning consent must be *Freely given, Reversible, Informed, Enthusiastic,* and *Specific.*[65] You may recall situations in your sexual history when you did not give consent and your *no* was violated or ignored. These recollections may be distressing. Be kind to yourself: you didn't know what you didn't know. It's true that we all do better when we know better.

To do better, you need to have an understanding of consent that is rock-solid. For that, we'll turn to the work of Dr. Betty Martin, a retired chiropractor and Certified Surrogate Partner. In the field of sexual education, she's known as an expert on consent. In fact, much of the information you'll find in this chapter is adapted directly from her work.[66] The dictionary defines *consent* as agreeing to something that somebody else wants, and one way to do that is to give permission.[67] Let's look at how Betty explains the difference between the two:

Consent is not the same as permission—it is far more than permission. If you hear other people saying, 'I give my consent,' what they actually mean is that they 'give their permission.' Permission means someone wants to do something and you are okay with it.

Think about the difference between 'wanting to' and 'willing to.' 'Willing to' is when someone else wants to do something and you're okay with it and you're willing to go along with it. 'Want to' is something that you want for your own reasons for yourself. When we're willing to have something done to us, we give permission. When we are wanting something, what we do is that we ask for what we want. Big difference. The cornerstone for the whole notion of consent is asking for what you want, which is a discipline, a challenge, a spiritual practice, and it's the road to freedom. The hardest thing about asking for what you want is knowing what you want. That's where it all has to start. We don't know how to ask for what we want. We need to take the time to figure out what we want.[68]

The first part of learning consent is figuring out what you honestly want. It's about gaining the ability to decisively say what you do and do not want regarding touch. This is particularly challenging for many women when it comes to sexuality. We've never been encouraged to discover what we want, which is precisely why we took you through all the pleasure practices in Parts I and II. Now that you're more in touch with your own desires, you can begin to share them with your partner, using consent as a communication tool.

There's great power in speaking your truth, whether it means saying *yes* or *no*. Stating *no* is nourishing to the nervous system, psyche, and soul. It's a muscle we all need to strengthen. *No* is a one-word sentence. By saying *no*, we take care of ourselves as well as others. Just think about it; when you are able to accept someone else's *no*, you'll more likely trust that when they say *yes*, they really mean it. Consent requires us to tune in to what our body wants and to use words that express those desires clearly. It also means setting our own limits and respecting those of others. Appropriate use of consent can change not only your relationship, but your whole life. Pause here and let that thought sink in.

Now you're ready for the meatier stuff. Let's begin by introducing you to the 3-Minute Game[69] which was created by Harry Faddis, professional life coach and spiritual director. He developed the game to help people ask for what they want in the present moment. Asking for what you want is the hardest and scariest part because most people don't really know what kind of touch they want. Playing the 3-Minute Game helps you figure out what you want as well as what you don't want. Basically, this is what happens in the game: you ask for some form of touch that you want, you get it, and you are grateful for it.

The game, played by two people, is based on two questions: "What do you want me to do to you?" and "What do you want to do to me?" Each partner negotiates their limits and never gives more than they are willing and happy to give. Both get the opportunity to ask for what they want and then receive three minutes of undivided attention.

Over time, Betty adapted and further developed the game. To better understand and conceptualize what was happening in the game, she created the Wheel of Consent.

The Wheel of Consent is probably new to you. As we describe it, go slowly through the material. We encourage you to spend a lot of time studying the slightly modified diagram below and soaking it in. There's a ton of good stuff going on here; it may take two or three readings before you're able to really wrap your head around what it means and to begin to apply it successfully.

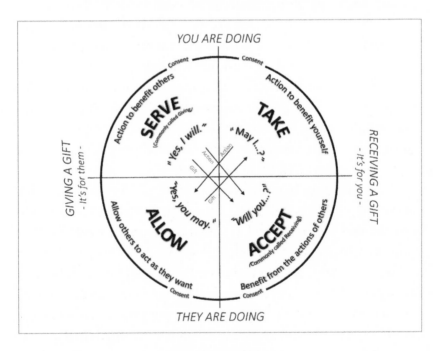

The Wheel of Consent
Adapted and published with permission from Betty Martin.

The Wheel of Consent divides consent into four activities and places them in separate quadrants: *Serve, Take, Accept,* and *Allow.* The axes divide the circle to define what *you are doing* or what *they are doing* and who the gift of pleasure is for (*it's for them* or *it's for you*). We'll first discuss the "doing" half and the activities that fall within it. Then we'll look at how each activity relates to consent. At the end of the chapter, you'll be given the prescriptions to help you and your partner practice consent, perhaps for the first time.

Before reading on, take a deep breath. As we've said, this is a huge topic. Consent is so important. The work it requires may bring up past trauma, resentment, and fear. It might even put a temporary strain on your relationship as you wrangle your way through it. It's okay to fumble. Practice it again and again. It holds so much promise. Deeper intimacy can develop when couples implement proper consent.

A Note from Elizabeth:

You may come up against a lot of old stuff when you start to work with consent. Many women only recently started thinking about these issues when they came into the public conversation through the #MeToo movement in 2017. Issues of trust and safety, or the lack thereof, may have resurfaced for you.

It shouldn't come as a huge surprise that some of the same issues may be coming up for the guy in your life. The rules of consent are new to everybody. We've all grown up living in a culture that discouraged women's sexual freedom, where consent was never part of the vocabulary. It's a game changer for everyone. So, as long as your partner is honestly trying, give him a break. Do your best to understand the concept of consent and go easy on him as you both go through the learning process together.

Don't be surprised to discover that he might not know what he wants. Be ready for that. You may find it useful to show him the resources that helped you in Chapters Five and Six. Once he understands more of what he does and does not want, it's my hope he too sees value in practicing consent in your relationship.

Solidly practicing consent in relationships is a deeply intimate experience. More often than not, a shift to a truly consensual relationship becomes permanent as both partners get more of their intimate needs met. We hope that this is true for you. In fact, we hope that you take it beyond touch itself and into your entire relationship.

But does the Wheel of Consent stop at touch and sex? Absolutely not! The four quadrants can also be used for nonsexual expression that contribute to your overall intimacy as a couple. Think of how often you willingly agreed to eat Thai food when you really wanted Italian. By eating Thai with your partner, you willingly served his pleasure. Or, let's say your partner needs to borrow your car to go have fun with his friends. You are happy to say yes but state a limit that he returns by 5 p.m. so you can drive it to dinner with your girlfriends. Working with consent is a natural part of any healthy relationship.

To really understand this, we'll break it down piece by piece. To start, let's look at just half of the Wheel of Consent.

When You Are Doing: Serve and Take

The two quadrants in the upper half of the Wheel of Consent involve the things you are doing.

A very simple way of looking at this is to understand who is doing the action. In this upper half, it's you. When in the Serve quadrant, you *serve* by doing something for your partner for *their* pleasure and benefit. For example, you might respond to your partner's request by saying, "Yes, I will touch you that way because it will bring you pleasure." If you're in the Take quadrant, you *take* by doing something to your partner because it brings *you* pleasure and benefit to do it. For example, you might say, "May I touch you this way because it will bring me pleasure?"

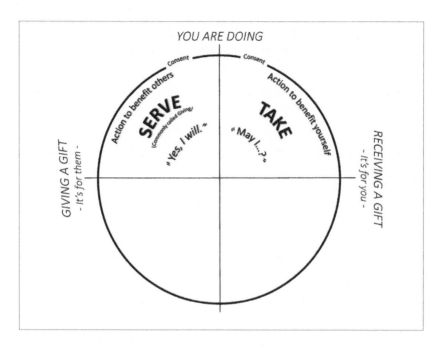

The "You Are Doing" half of the Wheel of Consent

To *serve* is commonly called *giving*. What you are giving is touch in the way that your partner requests; it's the gift you give as an action that benefits your partner. It's a little unusual in that you set aside what you want *and* you take responsibility for setting limits on what you are willing to give, as Betty says, "freely and with a full heart." Your partner asks, "Will you stroke my arm?" You respond, "Yes, I will stroke your arm, but just the left one for ten minutes."

In the Take quadrant, it is for your own pleasure; you touch your partner in ways that are pleasing to you. It's solely about your turn-on, which may feel odd and selfish at first. Consider it instead as owning what you want and asking for permission to do it. In this scenario, you would ask your partner, "May I explore your back?" because feeling their back would feel really good to your hands. To *take* is just a natural expression of our own pleasure.

Now it's time to look at the other half of the wheel, which is all about what happens when your partner is touching you.

When They Are Doing: Allow and Accept

The two quadrants in the lower half of the Wheel of Consent involve the things that your partner is doing to you.

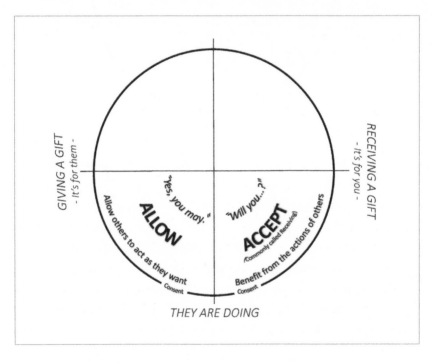

The "They Are Doing" half of the Wheel of Consent

On the bottom half, the roles are *allow* or *accept*. This is where you are when your partner is doing. From the Accept quadrant, you *accept* receiving something that you have requested for your pleasure or benefit. For example, you might have asked, "Will you touch me in this way for my pleasure?" When you are the Allow quadrant, you *allow* them to do something because it brings them pleasure and benefit. For example, you might respond to their request by saying, "Yes, you may touch me in the way you've requested for your pleasure."

To *accept* is commonly called *receiving*. This happens after you ask for a specific touch that you want and receive it from them for your pleasure. You are benefiting from their action; it's the gift of their touch that you are accepting. You ask, "Will you caress my face?" and then receive that caress.

To *allow* is to give your partner the gift of being able to touch you the way they want, but you set the boundaries for what you are willing to allow them to do. They have made a request, such as, "May I play with your chest?" And you have responded, "Yes, you may play with my chest as long as you don't squeeze my nipples." Basically, you give your partner permission to take pleasure from your body, but on your terms.

A Note from Dee:

Partners of women who are in pain are often in a terrible conundrum: they want her to have sexual pleasure, but they don't want to hurt her in the process. When touch or feeling arousal causes pain for her, some men end up just avoiding intimacy altogether.

In part, this is because many male partners of women with sexual pain just don't understand what's going on for their partner. I've heard this firsthand. After Elizabeth and I gave a talk about female sexual pain, one of the few men in the audience approached me during a break. He told me that his wife had pain with sex and he found our talk illuminating. For the first time, he understood what might be happening with his wife. "You need to talk to more men about this," he said passionately, "because we men really have no idea what's going on and how to deal with the pain." I agreed with him; men do need to know. I would suggest to any man in this situation that they read the first two chapters of this book to gain a better understanding.

At the same time, we need to have compassion and understand that this is hard for men too. Many men like to fix things and get things done. But here, neither of those tactics will work. As we've shown throughout this book, women have to address their pain with the assistance of compassionate health care providers as well as with the support from those who love them.

The Wheel of Consent can help with this. It's a really powerful tool for women with vulvar pain and their partners as they explore touch that is pleasing without doing further harm. It offers each person a way to consent and to "Serve," "Take," "Accept," and "Allow" touch in their relationship. What is most important to me is that it helps couples establish boundaries as they begin to explore sexuality with hope and excitement.

Although we talked about the wheel in two halves, in reality, things are often more fluid. To completely understand consent, each person (you and your partner) will, at some point, participate in the action represented in each of the four quadrants.

Let's look at how the four quadrants of the Wheel of Consent work together.

The Four Quadrants Together

Now that you know what each of the four quadrants are, it's time to play with them to fully experience all the different aspects of consent.

No matter which axis you use to split the Wheel of Consent—from You Are Doing to They Are Doing or from Giving a Gift (It's for Them) to Receiving a Gift (It's for You)—there may be positions on the wheel that feel easier or more difficult for you. What we have noticed is that the most difficult quadrants for people are *take* and *accept*, where the aspects of consent are solely about wanting to experience pleasure. This doesn't seem to be so for the partner who will either *serve* or *allow*, as it isn't about wanting pleasure, but about a willingness to *give* pleasure.

The difference between *want to do* and *willing to do* is a huge piece of grasping these concepts. When you *want to do* something, you do it for your own pleasure. When you are *willing to do something*, you do it to give someone else pleasure. The questions "May I?" or "Will you?" mean the person is asking for something that they want. The responses "Yes, you may" or "Yes, I will" indicate a willingness to do for that person what they have asked for. In the prescriptions, you'll have a chance to ask and answer all of these questions.

This is such a turnaround in regard to the way we've been taught to think about our own pleasure. Rather than focusing on our own needs, we spend time taking care of someone else's wants and needs. But actually, asking for the pleasure you want without having to give it in return is a wonderful gift you give to yourself. None of this can happen without knowing what you want. By the time you're this far in this book, you likely have a sense of the type of touch that brings you pleasure. This is your chance to explain, or guide, or show your partner what you've learned. Utilizing the Wheel of Consent will help you ask for whatever ignites your turn-on.

In thriving relationships where consent is being practiced, movement around the wheel is fluid. Couples cycle through the quadrants frequently, even in the same physical encounter; the process involves alternating between *serving/accepting* and *taking/allowing*. Once you understand that process and know how to operate within it, you're living the practice of consent full-on. Your intimate encounters will become more and more fulfilling.

On a practical level, this framework will help you develop the vocabulary you need to talk effectively about consent, exploring what you want and don't want as a team. On a deeper level, exploring the four quadrants can foster a sexy, intimate conversation about your most passionate desires. It takes the communication skills you used in Chapter Eight to a whole new level, one where you get the pleasure you want.

Now, let's look at the prescriptions. They can be done with your long-term partner or, like Leigh, explored with somebody new. In the first prescription, you and your partner will practice using the words *yes* and *no* while paying attention to how saying each feels in your body. We then move to a nonverbal game where both partners explore setting boundaries using hand gestures only. To end the chapter, we will bring the Wheel of Consent to life as you play the 3-Minute Game, exploring each of the four quadrants.

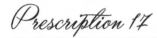

Prescription 17

The Impact of Saying Yes and No

The simplest and often most effective way to say *no* is to, well, say *no*! It may not always be easy. This exercise will help bring awareness to how your body responds when you say *no* in comparison to when you say *yes*.

What You'll Need:

- Thirty-plus minutes of complete, partnered privacy.

- A comfortable space.

- A pen and paper or a journal to record your reflections (optional).

Let's Get Started!

- Get comfortable and make sure you both understand the game before beginning.

- One partner asks the other a series of questions (see the list below), to which the other answers *no*.

- Both partners notice the sensations that come up in their body after each question and response.

- Be aware of the desire to apologize for a *no* even nonverbally. Stay present, even if it's awkward.

- Then, the same partner repeats the list of questions, with the other responding *yes*. Even though they answer *yes*, the point here is not to perform the actions; just let the *yes* hang in the air, and pay attention to how it feels.

- Switch roles and repeat the steps above.

- Partners may choose between quietly reflecting in silence or journaling about their experience, taking note of what was difficult, what was easy, and any bodily sensations they may have experienced. How did it feel to say *no* when you really wanted to say *yes*? How did it feel to say *yes* when you really wanted to say *no*? How did it feel to be told *no* ten times, or to have to say *no* over and over again?

- Then, each partner can take a turn and share their experience, using the listening skills you learned in Chapter Eight. Use this time to connect with each other.

- Here are some sample questions. Come up with your own. Be creative!

1. May I rub your shoulders?

2. Will you take your clothes off?

3. Will you hug me?

4. May I stick my finger up your nose?

Using Body Language to Convey Consent

Yes and *no* can be communicated nonverbally as well. Nonverbal communication is our first response; it comes even before we're able to find words to describe what's happening. That's because our bodies *feel* before we *think*; we react quicker than we respond. Because of that, nonverbal reactions are often more aligned with the emotional truth of a given situation. Our bodies sense and feel the difference between danger and safety, pleasure and pain, and avoidance and engagement.

What You'll Need:

- Thirty-plus minutes of complete, partnered privacy.

- A larger-sized room with space to walk.

- A pen and paper or a journal to record your reflections (optional).

Let's Get Started:

- Determine who will be the first to practice giving consent before beginning.

- Stand across the room from each other with a clear path between you.

- Partner A practices asking for Partner B to walk forward by holding up their hands and making one of three signs to match their desired level of closeness:

  ▸ *Come hither*:
    With your palm facing up, motion for your partner to

come toward you as if you were saying, "I want you to come closer."

▸ *Stop*:
Hold your arm straight in front of you, palm facing your partner, as if you were saying, "I want you to stay right there."

▸ *Back away*:
With your palm facing down, use your fingers to shoo them away, as if you were saying, "I want you to back away."

- Check in with your body and make the motions that feel most natural.

- While this is happening, Partner B moves forward and back exactly as motioned. Stay patient and compassionate in this role, and be aware of how it feels to receive your partner's requests.

- Partner A continues using the three hand signals until Partner B is standing in front of them at a distance that feels just right.

- Partner A clasps their hands together to end the exercise.

- Switch roles and repeat the steps above.

- Partners may choose between quietly reflecting or journaling about their experience, recording what was difficult, what was easy, and any bodily sensations they may have experienced. Notice what it felt like to ask for your own needs to be met, or to meet your partner's. Identify whether your comfort zone was vastly different from your partner's and note how that feels.

- Then, each partner can take a turn to share, using the listening skills you learned in Chapter Eight.

Prescription 19

The 3-Minute Game

You can download a small, printable booklet version of the 3-Minute Game on Betty's website in order to follow along with our directions below.[70] You will see that Betty's 3-Minute Game is different from the one Harry first created.

Betty's game is also based on two questions, each one an offer that is asked in this way:

- Offer #1: Partner A is in the Serve quadrant and asks, "How would you like me to touch you for three minutes?" Partner B is in the Accept quadrant and responds, "Will you…?" Partner A negotiates their limits and never gives more than they are happy to give, stating "Yes, I will," only when they're comfortable with the terms. The pair then engages in the negotiated touch for three minutes.

- Offer #2: Partner A while in the Allow quadrant asks, "How would you like to touch me for three minutes?" Partner B while in the Take quadrant responds, "May I…?" Partner A negotiates their limits and never gives more than they are happy to give, stating, "Yes, you may," and, as before, based on their agreed upon terms. The pair then engages in the negotiated touch for three minutes.

- Partner A and Partner B switch roles so that each has a turn making and responding to the offers.

As a reminder:

- To Serve: You are doing and it's for them

- To Take: You are doing and it's for you

- To Allow: They are doing and it's for them

- To Accept: They are doing and it's for you

Each quadrant presents its own challenges, lessons, and joys and will teach you something different about yourself.

What You'll Need:

- Thirty-plus minutes of complete, partnered privacy.

- A comfortable location with relaxing lighting, etc.

Let's Get Started:

- Get comfortable and make sure you both understand the game before beginning.

- Choose who will first make Offer #1 (Partner A) and who will respond (Partner B).

- Negotiate as needed until you find agreement or choose another offer.

- Start with nonsexual requests for touch.

- Then, set a timer for three minutes and fulfill the offer.

- It's okay to change your mind in the middle if you want something different or if you've had enough.

- Next, Partner A makes Offer #2 to Partner B.

- Negotiate as needed until you find agreement or choose another offer.

- Start with nonsexual requests for touch.

- Then, set a timer for three minutes and fulfill the offer.

- Partner A and Partner B switch roles so that each has a turn making and responding to the offers.

- At the end of the exercise, close it by thanking your partner.

<hr>

TIPS FOR EACH QUADRANT

To Serve

1. Set aside what you prefer (including the response you hope to see).

2. Ask what your partner wants—and wait for the answer. Making space for their choice is the most important part.

3. Decide if you are willing and able to do that. Honor your limits. Ask yourself: Is this something I can give with a full heart?

4. If it is, do so as best you can.

5. Say, "You're welcome!"

To Take

1. Ask your partner what their limits are and abide by them, completely.

2. Take the time to notice what part of them you would like to feel.

3. Ask "May I..." not "would you like..."

4. Use your hands to feel, not to serve. Move slowly; the slower you go, the more you feel. Feel for the shape and texture.

5. When you start trying to give to them, remind yourself it is for you.

6. Say, "Thank you!"

To Allow

1. Take time to consider your limits. Ask yourself: Is this a gift I can give with a full heart?

2. Wait for a resounding inner *yes!*

3. If you are hesitant, it's either because:

    ‣ You need more information—and if so, ask for it,

    ‣ It's a *no* waiting for you to hear it—and if so, say *no*, or

    ‣ If you set a certain limit, it would be a yes—and if so, ask yourself what that limit is.

4. Say, "You're welcome!"

To Accept

1. Put yourself first. Set aside what you are okay with. Go for wonderful.

2. Take the time you need to notice what it is you would like. This is the most important part, and often the hardest.

3. Ask as directly and specifically as you can. No hinting, no maybes, no whatever-you-want-to-give. Stop trying to give your giver a good experience. That's their job.

4. Change your mind at any time (ask for something different).

5. Say, "Thank you!"

Consent throughout the Relationship

Congratulations! You made your way through some of the most complex material in the book. Give yourself a pat on the back. At first, working with consent may seem difficult and confusing. Trust us, we get it! But two partners who really understand how *yes* and *no* feel in their bodies, and truly know what they want at any given time, have the potential to create a very intimate connection together. Consider Leigh; she and her new boyfriend worked with the consent prescriptions to develop a very different relationship than the one she'd had with her ex-husband. This time, she found the intimacy and pleasure that, deep down, she knew was hers to claim.

Consent greatly increases the degree of perceived safety people feel when connecting. It allows space for the same spontaneity and free expression between two people that you developed on your own in Parts I and II. Each partner learned that giving and receiving consent is vital to a thriving sexual connection. By communicating openly and exploring consent, you create a safe and supportive cushion for sexuality to flourish in your relationship. This is true of longstanding relationships, such as a marriage of several decades. It's also true of new relationships, such was the case of Leigh and her boyfriend. Using the Wheel of Consent and playing the 3-Minute Game, the couple built a lasting long-term relationship based on consent.

In the next chapter, we'll look at using your newfound skills of communication and consent to explore partnered touch. Through the prescriptions in this book, you've learned what works for you and what doesn't work; you've learned how to ignite your turn-on when you engage sexually in order to reduce your pain and increase your pleasure. It's time to bring your partner on board, inviting him to participate in your pleasure on a deeper level.

If you're aiming toward finding a pleasurable way to have penetrative sex, this next chapter is key; it's the ultimate step on your journey. Get ready to bring everything you have learned together as you play with joyful, wanted, pleasurable touch—together.

CHAPTER TEN

Exploring Partnered Touch

A Note from Dee:

> Gayle came to me with persistent low back pain. She was in
> her late fifties, had been married for over thirty years, and
> excitedly told me their youngest had just moved out. Gayle
> had been looking forward to "empty-nesting" as a time to find
> a deeper connection with her husband. Like all of my patients,
> her assessment included questions about her sex life. I asked
> her if her back pain limited her ability to enjoy sex. Gayle
> told me they had sex occasionally, but it wasn't all that great.
> To her, it seemed pretty matter of fact—in and out, and when
> he was finished, sex was over. The act itself didn't hurt, but it
> often made her back pain worse for a few days.
>
> When I asked her to clarify what "deeper connection"
> meant, she told me she wanted more affectionate touch, both
> inside and outside their bedroom. Gayle admitted she no
> longer reached out to her husband for hugs, kisses, or even
> to hold hands, as he took these gestures to mean she wanted
> sex. She shared that he had always been awkward with touch,
> even shying away from showing affection with their children.
> After thirty years of marriage, she wondered if any of this
> could be fixed. I told her I don't ever fix anybody, but I had
> tools that could help her fix their relationship.
>
> Gayle's first task was to work on easing her back pain. As
> part of my treatment plan, I gave her a prescription to explore

sensual pleasure, hoping to redirect her focus away from the back pain. At her follow-up several weeks later, she told me she'd followed my recommendations and that her back felt better. She'd found ways to include more sensuality in her days, stating it was quite nice and easy to do. Having spent time reconnecting to her sensual side, she was pleasantly surprised to realize she hadn't felt nearly as much pain and was anxious to hear what the next steps would be. By the end of that visit, Gayle was given additional treatments for her back pain as well as a new prescription that she and her husband could use together to begin a conversation about touch. Throughout her care, I prescribed strategies that she and her husband could use to let touch help deepen their connection, creating more intimacy in and out of the bedroom.

At her final appointment, Gayle said that when she used the tools I'd given her, her back pain was all but gone. Not only that, but her relationship with her husband had dramatically improved too. They were kissing, hugging, and touching more often. They had rediscovered an intimacy that hadn't been present since their early courtship, and Gayle laughed as she explained how much younger and more alive she felt. I can only imagine that her husband agreed: exploring partnered touch had changed their relationship for the better!

Gayle and her husband's relationship was quite common; there are a lot of couples who, for whatever reason, don't share affection regardless of how long they've been together. Some couples are perfectly okay with that, but Gayle wasn't. Many couples could benefit by upgrading the way they touch one another. In some cases, this is more of an up*date* as things may have once felt amazing. For both the upgrade and update to happen, a conversation about touch has to take place first. Many couples don't know how to talk about touch—sexual or otherwise. They may not know how to describe the type of touch they like, let alone feel comfortable asking for it. Chapter Nine gave you a great foundation in that you learned about consent and how to ask for, give, and get all kinds of touch. Now, we'll put that principle into action.

This chapter is about helping you and your partner learn how to touch each other in ways that feel good—like really good—by using nonsexual and sexual touch appropriately. Receiving touch that feels good requires you to know your body well and to state your desires. Like Gayle, you and your partner may need to relearn the nuance of touch from the ground up.

One of the many reasons to do so is that touch—whether it's sexual or not—is a major component of intimacy. Touch is also good for our health. We just plain *need* it. As Betty Martin told Elizabeth, "Touch is a human need that we're born with that never goes away, and it's absolutely essential for our well-being."[71]

Touch was critical to our development as children. Famous studies done on primates in the 1950s and 60s showed that, when facing frightening circumstances, infant monkeys turned to foam and soft terrycloth surrogate mothers seeking comfort. This pivotal research still stands today stressing the importance of comforting touch as a necessary building block in infant development and human behavior.[72] In the late 1980s, psychologists became aware of the effects of touch deprivation and other forms of child neglect on children raised in orphanages in Romania. By 1999, formal studies were launched to investigate how those effects impacted children long-term.[73] The research is ongoing, but the data show a clear pattern: many babies were not able to thrive in such an environment; among those living into adulthood, the psychological and physical effects are often long-lasting. Touch is very important for adults too. The difficulty is that we don't often understand how much we need touch, nor do we know how to get it safely and appropriately in order to meet our basic needs.

Our clients and patients repeatedly told us that this was true for them. They wanted the deep connection that comes with touch. Consider the physiological and biochemical changes our bodies undergo when we're touching or being touched by another. Touch decreases our heart rate and lowers our blood pressure. It decreases cortisol, leading to lower stress levels, and increases oxytocin, the "snuggle hormone."[74] These effects may be temporary, but in some cases, they're ongoing; the frequency of partner hugs has been linked to many of these effects over the long term.[75]

These physiological responses suggest that there's great safety in touch. In one study, brain scans of women taken while they were being threatening with electric shock showed their threat responses were less active when they were holding their husband's hand. What's more interesting is that when their relationship quality was rated higher, their threat responses were even less.[76]

Humans thrive from safe and loving touch. Simply put, good touch is good for us. Yet as adults in modern society, we often don't touch enough. In 2018, the *Guardian* asked whether people were touching too little, implying that the hypervigilant boundaries in the wake of the #MeToo movement created a "crisis of touch."[77] It's clear that #MeToo has done a lot of good in the world, yet plenty of people still stand to develop better skill sets around consent and communication. Others honestly want to do the right thing with touch, but are fearful, not knowing how to touch in ways that are appropriate and welcomed. In 2019, writer Mark Greene described the difficulty men face in the #MeToo era:

> Accordingly, it has become every man's job to prove they can be trusted, in each and every interaction, day by day and case by case. In part, because so many men have behaved poorly. And so, we prove our trustworthiness by foregoing physical touch completely in any context in which even the *slightest* doubt about our intentions might arise. Which, sadly, is pretty much every context we encounter.[78]

One of the best places for us to get our touch needs met, regardless of our gender, is through our relationship. Yet even in these relationships, finding a comfortable way to touch can be challenging. The trick is for us to find a way to touch others lovingly so that it is fully received, while also allowing ourselves to be touched in ways that are pleasurable to us. That takes time, patience, and likely many adjustments. It also includes understanding that we're not all coming from the same place; each one of us was raised differently and has a different relationship with touch.

This chapter first dives into touch backgrounds, looking at how our ideas around touch are formed. Then, we'll teach you a tried-and-true method you can both use to teach your partner the many ways you desire to be touched, which will help you expand your vocabulary around what you like and don't like. Finally, we'll look at how you can bring all of that together, along with what you learned about communication and consent in the previous chapters, to touch each other in ways that are deeply pleasurable. Keep reading; this chapter includes the final tools you need to enter the world of mind-blowing partnered pleasure.

Understanding Touch Backgrounds

We all come to an understanding of touch from different perspectives, having come from different backgrounds. Considering the culture and family we were raised in can teach us a lot about touch.

There are larger cultural factors, based on the part of the world we were raised in and how touch was particular to the societal mores of that culture. In some, displays of touch are forbidden and dangerous; in others, touch is openly shared. On the familial level, the way touch was navigated—whether it was offered or withheld, accepted or admonished—in the house where you grew up impacts how you engage with touch as an adult. What you saw, what you heard, how you were touched or not, and how you were or weren't encouraged to touch those you loved are all determinants of the type of touch household in which you were raised. We form our behaviors and attitudes surrounding touch based on our touch household. Then over time, we experience touch in varying situations that either back up or alter our behaviors and attitudes.

As Gayle and her husband came to discover, the touch households they were raised in were quite different from each other. Gayle was raised in a house with loving and affectionate touch, while her husband grew up in a house where touch was almost nonexistent.

Our touch background contributes to our understanding of what's appropriate and what isn't, and in some cases, this leads to confusion. For example, if you grew up seeing your dad hit your mom, you may have thought, as a child, it was an okay thing to do. With maturity, such behavior is recognized as inappropriate. It used to be appropriate for a therapist or doctor to reach out and touch a patient while delivering difficult news; now, all they can offer is a box of tissues. The line between appropriate and inappropriate touch seems to be in constant flux, sometimes shifting very quickly like we saw in response to #MeToo and the COVID-19 pandemic, which created worldwide fear and confusion around touch overnight. As a global culture, it is yet to be seen how these events will shift our understanding of appropriate and inappropriate touch going forward.

Finding a shared definition for appropriate touch may be easier with a broader perspective. *We consider touch to be "appropriate" when it's contextual, consensual, and contractual.* In addition, the act must be warranted by the situation. It's appropriate for a hairdresser to wash your hair, while it wouldn't be for your dentist to do it. Though it is appropriate for your hairdresser to wash your hair, it isn't appropriate for him to wash your armpits. Appropriate forms of touch include touch that is therapeutic, healing, comforting, or nurturing when used in the proper context.

It's way easier to define what inappropriate touch is. Any touch that is uninvited, unwelcomed, or initiated without consent is inappropriate. It's also super helpful to know the intent of the touch.

Getting clear about your own intention and whether the touch is *for you* or *for them*, can help. One's intent behind touch can be *to give, to get, to console, to arouse,* or *to relax,* etc. Understanding everyone's intent makes room for you and others to invite, welcome, and initiate appropriate touch.

Your upbringing and the context in which you were raised also taught you what you know about sexual and nonsexual touch. Sexual touch is meant to excite, arouse, build pleasure, and increase turn-on. It seems as though the difference between that and non-sexual touch should be clear-cut but, unfortunately, that's not often the case. Touch isn't a subject matter taught in any school we know of. Instead, young people, old people, singles, and couples are left to figure it out for themselves. Let's face it, touch is inherently arousing. And what we mean by that is that when we physically touch someone somewhere on their body, we awaken or "arouse" that part of the body to a new feeling of sensation. Using that definition, hopefully you'll see that while all touch is arousing, it doesn't mean that all touch is *sexually* arousing.

Remember when we talked about the intent of touch? A mother reaching out for her daughter's hand with the intent of comforting her child is an example of nonsexual touch. A husband who holds his wife in a soothing embrace after a difficult day is another. Too often, however, the intent of nonsexual touch is misconstrued as sexual or erotic. Because of this, many of our clients told us that they had stopped touching altogether; they'd become touch avoidant.

Touch avoidance is a big issue. We believe the US is in a touch crisis as one of the least touched societies in the world. Somehow, we've lost the ability to get our basic touch needs met; we don't know how to touch, how to ask for touch, or even acknowledge that we need it. We've also forgotten how important regular, caring, nonsexual touch is for our health in general. The many benefits of touch are well documented and include the following:

- Reduces heart rate

- Regulates breathing

- Calms the central nervous system

- Releases oxytocin and other feel good hormones

- Improves bonding

- Acts as an analgesic

- Reduces depression and anxiety

The more positive experiences we create with our partners around nonsexual touch, the greater the likelihood that we'll move into pleasurable sexual touch.

Armed with this information, you and your partner can identify your touch backgrounds. You are now able to differentiate sexual from nonsexual touch and have a better understanding of what forms of touch are appropriate and inappropriate. *Voilà*, your touch skills have already improved. From here, we'll move on to teach you the many different types of touch you can use together.

Types of Touch

There are many types of touch and many ways to go about touching. Each one is important, as many factors go into the type of touch that we enjoy. It's unusual that any two people enjoy the exact same type of touch.

We touch in many different ways: pressing, pinching, caressing, stroking, tapping, and scratching are all potentially pleasurable ways to touch. The pressure with which we touch, whether we use a lot or a little, can make or break our partner's pleasure. People like wildly different pressures, often at different times, and sometimes just the variance of pressure is arousing. The length of strokes can go from long, full-bodied strokes to short ones over a specific area.

We can touch using a variety of speeds, from quick, fast strokes to slow, drawn-out caresses. In general, though, we always suggest touching your partner more slowly than you think you should; research consistently shows that people prefer slow touch, and often the slower the better.[79]

A Note From Dee:

Even without formal bodywork training, we can do a lot of good by working with the lymphatic system. Light lymphatic touch *is a very clinical way to describe the slow, sweeping, surface-level movements people often make when comforting each other. You know the type; it's that sort of light, open-palmed caress you might give to a child at bedtime, or the way you might soothe someone who has just received bad news by running your hand up and down their arm.*

This technique helps move the lymph, *a fluid that both carries white blood cells around the body to fight infection and helps remove wastes and toxins. Lymph runs in channels that lie just under the surface of the skin. In addition, manipulating the lymph can also help decrease inflammation and boost the immune system. When done by a trained therapist, this gentle technique is called* lymphatic drainage *or* lymph massage. *I believe some of the same benefits can be derived from receiving simple, sweet, light massaging touch; this type of touch not only feels good, it's beneficial for your health!*

This type of light touch can have mental health benefits too; it tells our nervous system that it's safe to relax, improving mood and sleep, and is generally helpful when we're feeling out of sorts. It's enjoyable to give and to receive. You can experiment with rhythms and speeds, all done with that super-light pressure, gentle enough to move only the surface of the skin. Every bit of it will benefit you and your partner's health and well-being.

One way to think of these types of touch is to consider them in terms of the four elements: earth, air, fire, and water. *Earth touch* is grounding, slow, with moderate to heavy amounts of pressure. *Air touch* is light and quick, involving swift, sometimes barely there movement with just a small amount of pressure. *Water touch* varies in speed, but its steady pressure is always fluid, continuous, curving over the body or arriving in waves. *Fire touch* is erratic, moves everywhere, and generates a lot of heat.

As you explore touch with your partner, notice what aspects draw you in. You may find yourself gravitating toward one of these elements and identifying which types of touch increase your arousal on the Pleasure Calibration Scale™. Make note of these things and share them with your partner. Keep the lines of communication open. Be as descriptive as possible.

Because the type of touch you enjoy can be affected by one or more of the influencers affecting your sexual core, know that this will be an ongoing conversation. The type of touch you desire can change from day to day or even within the course of a single encounter.

A number of factors impact the type of touch a woman might want. Her hormones can have a significant effect on how she experiences touch. For instance, some women experience breast tenderness when they're premenstrual; others don't want to be touched when they're nursing. Postmenopausal women, who have lost most of their subcutaneous fat, may want a gentler touch. In addition, physical traumas such as injuries, surgeries, and other medical interventions can change how we experience and appreciate touch. Factors like reaching adequate arousal levels, producing enough lubrication, and the absence or presence of pain can also contribute to what type of touch you prefer.

As these factors arise, utilize positive communication and the Wheel of Consent to convey the types of touch that would feel the best for you.

Expanding Partnered Experiences

As you start incorporating more intimate touch in your partnership, it may dawn on you that this is the first time in years that you've explored touch together. The thought of it might be frightening and foreign, but you have plenty of tools to help you achieve success. Remember the breathing exercises in Chapter Two? Do them together! Take this at your own pace; experiment by slowing down and tuning in to what feels good. Communicate, communicate, communicate!

A Note from Elizabeth:

Whenever I talk to couples about what it's like when they're intimate, I ask each of them how well they give and receive feedback about how things feel. To get the most benefit out of partnered touch, couples need to be able to do both well. Most of them had no idea how to tell their partner that what they were doing wasn't working; they responded with some version of "I don't want to hurt their feelings, so I just don't say anything." On the flip side, even when they thought they were doing what their partner liked, they felt rejected when they found out otherwise. This happens all too frequently and is unfortunate because giving and receiving clear feedback is a loving and kind way for couples to get what they want from each other.

To make this happen, we have to create a feedback loop that builds rapport and fosters intimacy. It's important to have an ongoing conversation taking place in the moment while the touch is occurring. When something isn't working, I teach my clients to start by saying something positive, then request a change, and when the touch is pleasing, close the loop with praise.

It breaks down like this:

First, note what is working. "Mmmm, I love feeling close to you," you might say, or "I like it when you use your nails on my back." Or express how something is working: "It turns me on feeling you naked next to me," or "I get goosebumps down my spine when you use your tongue."

And then request a change away from something that isn't working: "Can you move your hand down a bit and apply more pressure?" or "Would you dig your nails in just a little deeper?" Make the request as specific as possible, even showing them what you want. If they are willing and make the change, thank them with either a well-timed moan, a sincere "thank-you," a kiss, or a gentle arm squeeze. Keep going until the desired outcome is reached. Honest appreciation goes a long way here, especially if the adjustment process takes a few rounds. Keep giving feedback that you appreciate their understanding and desire to give you pleasure. If your turn-on is building, be sure to let your partner know.

When you both utilize this feedback loop, it's a win-win!

This is a process, and it's all about exploration. Don't expect to be perfect and get everything right the first time. You're going to make mistakes; be gentle and move through them together. Don't forget to set the mood and emphasize all of the senses. If it's not clear, incorporating 24/7 foreplay is a great lead-in to these experiences. We hope by now you realize that in order to have pleasure you must be able to have fun. Go out and play!

Rather than tossing you into the deep end of the pool without a life preserver, we're going to inch you into deeper waters using a tried-and-true method that we've both used successfully for years: sensate focus. The method was developed to help couples be present and mindful of sensations moment by moment, rather than forcing pleasure and arousal. The process allows couples to move toward the intimacy they desire rather than bow to the pressure to reach a certain goal.

We'll be using a modified version of sensate focus to help you explore what you want with touch. What's needed is an open mind and willingness to become more acquainted with each other's body. There's no room for judgment as you observe what's happening in your body. Your job is to be present and simply notice what you feel.

When we implement the feedback loop and play with sensate focus, our experiences become more intimate and pleasurable. This ultimately leads to higher arousal and, you guessed it, better sex! By the end of this chapter, you'll be in the swim and hopefully getting it on with your partner.

The prescriptions that follow are the last we have to offer you. They will help expand your partnered-touch practice. By the final prescription, we hope your hearts will be thumping at the prospect of humping and that you'll be jumping at the chance to take your sex life through the roof!

Prescription 20

Identify Your Touch Household

By looking back at the environment in which you were raised, you have an opportunity to better understand how and why you touch the way you do. This exercise will help you identify the dynamics of touch present in your childhood home. Those dynamics set the template for how you touch as an adult.

Be present for any emotions that arise, without making excuses for them. The goal is not about changing the past, but rather finding a way to understand the impact it has had. Be patient, take your time, and record your findings.

What You'll Need:

- At least thirty minutes of relative privacy in a comfortable place.

- A journal and a pen.

Let's Get Started!

- Sit quietly and think back to your childhood. Recall your parents, siblings, and any other adults or children who were involved in raising you.

- Consider how each of them demonstrated touch.

- Then, answer the following questions in your journal:

  ▸ Were you touched as a child? If so, who touched you? How and when did you feel comfortable being touched? Was it appropriate: kind, affectionate, and loving? Was it inappropriate: rough, tough, or abusive? Was there enough of it or too much?

  ▸ What touch did you witness between adults and other children? Was it appropriate: kind, affectionate, and loving? Was it inappropriate: rough, tough, or abusive? Was there enough of it or too much?

  ▸ What touch did you witness among other children? Was it appropriate: kind, affectionate, and loving? Was it inappropriate: rough, tough, or abusive? Was there enough of it or too much?

  ▸ What touch did you witness between adults? Was it appropriate: kind, affectionate, and loving? Was it inappropriate: rough, tough, or abusive? Was there enough of it or too much?

  ▸ Did you touch anyone? If so, who did you touch? How and when did you feel comfortable touching? Was it appropriate: kind, affectionate, and loving? Was it inappropriate: rough, tough, or abusive? Was there enough of it or too much?

- When you've finished writing, take a moment to reflect on

what you've written.

- Be gentle and consider any feelings and sensations that arise.

- If negative sensations arise, know you're safe now. Breathe, stretch, or take a short walk.

- Let this information land solidly in your body.

- When you're ready, talk to your partner. Share with them what you learned about your touch household.

- Ask your partner to complete this exercise, and when they are ready, talk about it with you.

- If any part of this exercise triggered painful or disturbing memories, please seek professional counseling.

Prescription 21

Putting It Together with Your Partner— Level 1

In this exercise, you and your partner will explore touching each other in a variety of ways, identifying what feels best, without touching genitals (no nipples, breasts, vulvas, or even penises). In Level 1, you are asked to stay away from penetration and orgasms; we like to refer to this as "outercourse." Remember, you need an open mind and the willingness to become more acquainted with each other's body. The goal is to be present; there's no need to strive toward a specific destination. To get the most out of this experience, go slowly and enjoy the pleasure. We recommend that you both are naked.

What You'll Need:

- Forty-five-plus minutes of complete, partnered privacy.

- A comfortable, warm, sensually pleasing environment. For most couples, the bedroom is the best place to use this prescription. Include music, lighting, and scents to enhance the space.

- A timer.

- Optional: Massage oil.

Let's Get Started!

- To start, identify which roles you will each take. Partner A will be the "toucher"; Partner B, the "receiver."

- Set the timer for fifteen minutes to start.

- Adhere to the guidelines set forth. Use all the time allowed; no more, no less.

- Throughout the experience, Partner B should use the feedback loop to address anything that feels uncomfortable.

- Partner A starts the timer as they begin to explore Partner B's body. Start with the extremities and work your way toward the center of Partner B's body. Touch their hands, arms, feet, scalp, and face. Try different types of touch, such as the ones described earlier.

- As you go through this exercise, remember it's an exploration to discover what feels good.

- When the timer goes off, switch roles and repeat each step.

- We encourage you to enjoy talking, hugging, and kissing throughout.

- Once you've both had a turn, share what it felt like.

- End the time by thanking each other.

Welcome to the Pleasure Movement

ongratulations! You are now part of the Pleasure Movement™!
The last ten chapters led you through a truly revolutionary
process. We live in a culture that tells us women don't deserve
pleasure and yet you bucked all convention to find yours. That is
no small feat; we are highly impressed!

Looking Back on this Book

Throughout the course of this book, you've learned an incredible
amount about yourself. You've learned the ins and outs of your
anatomy, exploring how to optimize your arousal network and the
functions it serves. We've deeply explored how pain works and how
pleasure might serve to heal it. We've offered you ways to better
connect to your sensual experience of the world around you. And
you've explored multiple types of touch and how to use them to
increase your sensual pleasure.

Then, you identified the influencers currently affecting your
ability to access your sexuality, part of an ongoing practice as your
influencers change. You began to do the deep, rewarding work of
looking at your sexual core, considering your unique body, turn-on,
and choice of sexual expression. We walked you through opening
your body to pleasurable penetration.

With your partner, you went deep into communication techniques to improve your whole relationship. You explored consent,

finding new ways to connect with your desire and ask for what you want. We led you through touching each other, slowly and methodically, with the aim of bringing you back toward pleasurable penetrative sex.

If, in the process, you managed to significantly reduce or even fully rewire your experience with sexual pain, *brava*! We bet you're jumping for joy! And if the changes are still coming, we hope that the stronger understanding of what's going on and the larger vocabulary to describe it can help you work with both your partner and your medical professional to address it. We hope that you understand that pain is not your fault, and that you have a newfound confidence about your sexual experience that will help you to explain what is happening and get the help you need.

But that wasn't our only aim—not by a long shot! The truth is, we hope this book has done a whole lot more than bring pleasure back into your sexual relationship; we hope it enhanced your experience of pleasure *throughout your entire life*.

From Overcoming Pain to Living a Pleasure-Forward Life

We've seen it happen; we've seen many women expand their experience of pleasure as their pain diminished. In these pages, you met ten of them. Some of their symptoms may have matched yours, while others weren't part of your reality. The stories of these ten women represent the most common problem-and-solution profiles we have seen over the course of our careers.

Jaime, Susana, Laura, Mary, Tara, Sarah, Danielle, Amanda, Leigh, and Gayle are all different in fundamental ways. Some were older, some younger. Some were partnered for years, while others were single. Some had children and others did not. They all had varying degrees of pain, likely with a different set of causes. Yet for all of them, the basic prescription was the same: each of these women learned how to get back in touch with her pleasure.

Yet none of these women were healed with a single prescription; in fact, over time, many of these women received quite a few pleasure prescriptions. In all cases, these pleasure prescriptions became part of a greater lifestyle shift. These ten women learned to check in with their bodies on a regular basis, creating a more sensual way of moving through their lives. They learned how to touch themselves and their partners to increase desire as part of the unique recipe to improve their turn-on. They learned to work through their pain by increasing their pleasure. And in all cases, these women expressed that the prescriptions we offered significantly improved their lives.

The greater promise of this book is that you create a life that is truly pleasure-forward. We want you to live an optimal life, one that's fueled by pleasure. We want you to consider what feels good with every step you take, from the first sip of coffee in the morning to the moment you fall asleep at night. We want you to create a healthy, amazing new relationship with your body as it soaks in pleasure.

The ten women you met in this book discovered that pleasure is their birthright and never looked back. We hope that you, too, are able to create that lifestyle shift. By this point, you've had plenty of opportunity to learn that pleasure heals. The rewards are immediate. So *don't stop.* Keep using the prescriptions, exploring your pleasure on a deeper and deeper level. Keep learning about yourself!

Doing so will help you thrive as a sexual being. It will move any standard black-and-white reality into Technicolor, guaranteed. Everyone will benefit as you live a pleasure-forward life. Think of yourself as a *Pleasure Ambassador*™. We are Pleasure Ambassadors. Come join us!

Becoming a Pleasure Ambassador

Hold on—you're probably asking what it means to be a Pleasure Ambassador. A *Pleasure Ambassador* is a person who is in touch with her own pleasure, lives a pleasure-forward life, and advocates pleasure for others. Not only does a Pleasure Ambassador have full sexual agency, but she wants it for everyone else, too, and she makes that part of her personal mission.

The symptoms of a pleasure-forward life vary from woman to woman. You may have noticed that you drink less coffee, need less sleep, or are more creative. You may feel more alive or alert. You may look sexier, you may laugh more freely, and, gosh darn it, you may just be happier. One thing's for sure: if you're living a pleasure-forward life, *people are going to notice and will want to know your secret.* We'd just love it if you answer honestly and fill them in on the details. Don't hold back; you know the truth.

Now, obviously there are right and wrong ways to go about sharing your story. If you're in the grocery store, it may not be well-received to explain in great detail what you learned from working on your own with a vibrator; if you're at the soccer field, it may not be the moment to share the specifics of how you and your partner took it through the roof. At the same time, pleasure is not selfish, nor is it a dirty word. It's part of overall wellness. And because of that, this stuff shouldn't be kept secret. Find your own way to spread this information far and wide. Whether you talk about sexual pleasure explicitly or in sly innuendos is up to you. Now, it's time for you to help other women learn about their own power.

Accessing pleasure is healthy. It's the fountain of youth! Pleasure strengthens our immune systems, keeping us younger and healthier both mentally and physically. It's an elixir of life-force (remember, Elizabeth says that orgasm is the world's first super-food!) that makes us happier, more joyful people. We want more healthy and well-pleasured people in the world. Pleasure is

A big thanks goes to our five fabulous kids—Jacob, Caleb, Nathan, Lucas, and Abbey—for tolerating the pelvic model that lived on our kitchen counter for years. You were all well versed in telling your friends what it was, even though none of them really wanted to know.

I want to thank my parents for teaching me that couples never argue in public, and parents should always present a united front when dealing with their kids. And last but certainly not least, my heartfelt thanks to my mother-in-law, Glenna, whose loving, caring, and undying support taught me that life was much more about kindness and understanding than bitterness and anger. These gifts together provide my life with immense joy and pleasure every day.

What would I do without Elizabeth Wood, my fellow partner-in-crime, sexuality soulmate, and creative co-author? Thank you, Elizabeth, for changing my life for the better, by bringing your own type of energy, cheekiness, knowledge, and experience to the table as we started our journey together. Who knew that the short time we spent together would create an unending friendship and affinity based on pain and pleasure? Without your talent, patience, and spirit, this book would never have come to fruition.

And lastly, I would like to extend a huge shout-out and thanks to the International Society for the Study of Vulvovaginal Disease (ISSVD). Though I'm appreciative of Howard Glazer's introduction to the ISSVD, I extend a huge thank-you to the entire society for welcoming me into your ranks, inviting me to present my work to audiences around the world, and (mostly) trusting that I wasn't from Mars. Your accolades for the benefits of physical therapy for women with chronic vulvar pain will forever give me pride and warm my heart.

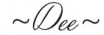

~Dee~

I would like to first thank my parents for always reminding me to "remember who you are." Turns out I'm someone who likes to talk about things that others don't, especially when it comes to sex! Next, I would like to offer Dan Powers boatloads of thanks for all the love and patience it took to be married to me throughout the rather lengthy writing process. You were there with hugs, regardless of how often I'd interrupt you in a panic over my IT needs. Thank you for giving me space so I could write the book and for sharing space with me when I wasn't.

To my amazingly talented co-author Dee Hartmann, thanks for letting me pluck you from retirement so that we could leave the legacy of our work on these pages. Without your gifts, talents, generosity of spirit, kindness, and time none of this would have happened. There are not enough words to express my profound gratitude for the special kinship we have, Dee.

Thanks to my sisters Jennifer Fithian and Margaret Whiting, who, with wonder and amazement, let me lift my wedding dress to show you mine and in return showed us yours. To Charlotte Muzik, who, although you missed that reveal, was present for so many other hilarious activities that we four Wood girls experienced together.

To my three nieces, Jessica Williamson and Marie and Joanna Fithian, and my five nephews, Drew Fithian, Oliver and William Whiting, and Bennet and Avery Robbins, who tolerate Crazy Aunt Lizzie. You love me even though I send you sex-positive educational books, tuck tubes of lubricant into your honeymoon suitcase, and remind you I am here to answer any question you might have. It's my hope that you will always make the most informed, pleasure-forward decisions, thrive in your relationships, and have healthy, wonderful sex lives.

To Kristin Viken, Elizabeth Mayne, Karen Krauss, and the Deer Tribe Metis Medicine Society for your encouragement, support, and trust, I thank you. I am honored to be a student of and to have been granted permission to share such revered teachings.

Thank you Jaiya for being such an inspiration and role model. You set the bar high for the betterment of all who desire high-quality sexuality education taught by persons with impeccable integrity.

And my thanks to Jennifer Molde and Terra Anderson for your graceful and thoughtful care in helping me better navigate LGBTQ+ terms and language.

~Elizabeth~

Endnotes

Chapter 1

1. Andrea Burri, Joceline Buchmeier, and Hartmut Porst, "The Importance of Male Ejaculation for Female Sexual Satisfaction and Function," *The Journal of Sexual Medicine* 15, no. 11 (November 2018): 1600–08.

2. Sheri Winston, *Women's Anatomy of Arousal: Secret Maps to Buried Pleasure* (Kingston, New York: Mango Garden Press, 2010).

3. Laura Fay, "Just 24 States Mandate Sex Education for K–12 Students, and Only 9 Require Any Discussion of Consent. See How Your State Stacks Up," *The 74*, April 1, 2019, https://www.the74million.org/article/just-24-states-mandate-sex-education-for-k-12-students-and-only-9-require-any-discussion-of-consent-see-how-your-state-stacks-up/.

4. Jennifer Knudtson and Jessica E. McLaughlin, "Female External Genital Organs," April 2019, https://www.merckmanuals.com/home/women-s-health-issues/biology-of-the-female-reproductive-system/female-external-genital-organs.

5. Knudtson and McLaughlin, "Female External Genital Organs."

6. Knudtson and McLaughlin, "Female External Genital Organs."

7. P. Polácek and L. Malinovský, "Fine Structure of the Sensory Nerve Endings in the Clitoris," *Zeitschrift fur mikroskopisch-anatomische Forschung* 84, no. 2 (December 1970): 293–310; M. Kantner, "Studies on the Sensory System of the Glans

Clitoridis," *Zeitschrift fur mikroskopisch-anatomische Forschung* 60, no. 3 (December 1953): 388–98.

8. Helen E. O'Connell, John M. Hutson, Colin R. Anderson, and Robert J. Plenter, "Anatomical Relationship between Urethra and Clitoris," *The Journal of Urology* 159, no. 6 (June 1998): 1892–1897, https://doi.org/10.1016/S0022-5347(01)63188-4.

9. Andrea Stanley and Sascha de Gersdorff (editors), "G-Spot Not Real," *Cosmopolitan Magazine*, April 7, 2020, https://www.cosmopolitan.com/interactive/a32037401/g-spot-not-real/.

10. Debra Herbenick and Michael Reece, "Development and Validation of the Female Genital Self-Image Scale," *The Journal of Sexual Medicine* 7, no. 5 (May 2010): 1822–30.

11. Natalie Amos and Marita McCabe, "Positive Perceptions of Genital Appearance and Feeling Sexually Attractive: Is It a Matter of Sexual Esteem?" *Archives of Sexual Behavior* 45, no. 5 (July 2016): 1249–58.

12. Vanessa R. Schick, Sarah K. Calabrese, Brandi N. Rima, and Alyssa N. Zucker, "Genital Appearance Dissatisfaction: Implications for Women's Genital Image Self-Consciousness, Sexual Esteem, Sexual Satisfaction, and Sexual Risk," *Psychology of Women Quarterly* 34, no. 3 (September 2010): 294–404.

13. National Institutes of Health National Cancer Institute, "Surveillance, Epidemiology, and End Results Program," 2019, https://seer.cancer.gov/statfacts/html/vulva.html.

Chapter 2

14. "Frequently Asked Questions: When Sex Is Painful," *The American College of Obstetricians and Gynecologists* (September 2017), https://www.acog.org/-/media/For-Patients/faq020.pdf.

15. Jenn Mann, "Why Sex Hurts," *InStyle Magazine*, August 30,

2018, https://www.instyle.com/lifestyle/why-sex-hurts.

16. Lili Loofbourow, "The Female Price of Male Pleasure," *The Week*, January 25, 2018, https://theweek.com/articles/749978/female-price-male-pleasure.

17. "Frequently Asked Questions: When Sex Is Painful," *The American College of Obstetricians and Gynecologists* (September 2017), https://www.acog.org/-/media/For-Patients/faq020.pdf.

18. Judith M. Schlaeger, et al., "Sensory Pain Characteristics of Vulvodynia and Their Association with Nociceptive and Neuropathic Pain: An Online Survey Pilot Study," *PAIN Reports* 4, no. 2 (February 2019): https://doi.org/10.1097/PR9.0000000000000713.

19. Sourced and adapted with permission from www.My-MS.org and James Jacobsen.

20. "NIH Research Plan on Vulvodynia," *US Department of Health and Human Services, National Institutes of Health, Eunice Kennedy Shriver National Institute of Health and Human Development* (April 2012), https://www.nva.org/wp-content/uploads/2015/01/NIH_Vulvodynia_Plan_April2012.pdf.

21. "Frequently Asked Questions: Vulvodynia," *The American College of Obstetricians and Gynecologists* (April 2017), https://www.acog.org/Patients/FAQs/Vulvodynia.

22. "Frequently Asked Questions: When Sex Is Painful," *The American College of Obstetricians and Gynecologists* (September 2017), https://www.acog.org/-/media/For-Patients/faq020.pdf.

23. "Vulvodynia: Get the Facts," *National Vulvodynia Association*, 2019, https://www.nva.org/media-center/.

24. D. S. Solursh, et al., "The Human Sexuality Education of Physicians in North American Medical Schools," *International Journal of Impotence Research* 15, no. S5 (2003): S41.

25. Courtney Ackerman, "What Is Neuroplasticity? A Psychologist Explains," *PositivePsychology*, July 25, 2018, https://positivepsychologyprogram.com/neuroplasticity/.

26. Beverly Whipple and Barry R. Komisaruk, "Analgesia Produced in Women by Genital Self-Stimulation," *The Journal of Sex Research* 24, no. 1 (January 1988): 130–40, https://doi.org/10.1080/00224498809551403.

27. Sheri Winston, *Women's Anatomy of Arousal: Secret Maps to Buried Pleasure* (Kingston, New York: Mango Garden Press, 2010).

28. Tammy Worth, "Does Vagina Size Matter?," *WebMD*, https://www.webmd.com/women/features/vagina-size#1.

29. Jamie Eske, "What to Know about Hormones," *Medical News Today*, April 4, 2019, https://www.medicalnewstoday.com/articles/324887.php.

Chapter 3

30. Michelle Roberts, "Scan Spots Women Faking Orgasms," *BBC News*, June 20, 2005, http://news.bbc.co.uk/2/hi/health/4111360.stm.

31. Resnick, Stella. "The ABC's of Pleasure," February 20, 2020, https://www.drstellaresnick.com/post/the-abc-s-of-pleasure.

Chapter 4

32. The Global Advisory Board on Sexual Health and Wellbeing, "Working Definition of Sexual Pleasure," 2016, https://www.gab-shw.org/our-work/working-definition-of-sexual-pleasure/.

33. *EtymoloGeek*, https://etymologeek.com/eng/masturbate; *Merriam-Webster*, https://www.merriam-webster.com/dictionary/self-abuse.

34. Domeena Renshaw, personal correspondence, Maywood, IL, 1997.

35. James G. Pfaus, Gonzalo R. Quintana, Conall Mac Cionnaith, and Mayte Parada, "The Whole versus the Sum of Some of the Parts: Toward Resolving the Apparent Controversy of Clitoral versus Vaginal Orgasms," *Socioaffective Neuroscience & Psychology* 6, no. 1 (2016): 32578, http://dx.doi.org/10.3402/snp.v6.32578.

36. James G. Pfaus, Gonzalo R. Quintana, Conall Mac Cionnaith, and Mayte Parada, "The Whole versus the Sum of Some of the Parts: Toward Resolving the Apparent Controversy of Clitoral Versus Vaginal Orgasms," *Socioaffective Neuroscience & Psychology* 6, no. 1 (2016): 32578, http://dx.doi.org/10.3402/snp.v6.32578.

37. Cindy M. Meston, et al., "Women's Orgasm," *Kinsey Institute*, https://kinseyinstitute.org/pdf/womens%20orgasm%20 annual%20review.pdf.

38. Cindy M. Meston, et al., "Women's Orgasm," *Kinsey Institute*, https://kinseyinstitute.org/pdf/womens%20orgasm%20 annual%20review.pdf.

39. James McIntosh, "Everything You Need to Know about Orgasms," *Medical News Today,* November 23, 2018, https:// www.medicalnewstoday.com/articles/232318.php.

40. Debby Herbenick, Tsung-Chieh (Jane) Fu, Jennifer Arter, Stephanie A. Sanders, and Brian Dodge, "Women's Experiences with Genital Touching, Sexual Pleasure, and Orgasm: Results from a U.S. Probability Sample of Women Ages 18 to 94," *Journal of Sex and Marital Therapy* 44, no. 2 (February 2018): 201–12. https://doi.org/10.1080/0092623X.2017.1346530.

41. *Merriam–Webster*, https://www.merriam-webster.com/dictionary/orgasm.

42. Valerie Morin, Sylvie Levesque, and Julie Lavigne, "Female Masturbatory Practices and Sexual Health: A Qualitative Exploration of Women's Perspectives," *Journal of Sexual Medicine* 14, no. 5 (May 2017): e270.

Chapter 5

43. Marie S. Carmichael, Richard Humbert, Jean Dixen, Glenn Palmisano, Walter Greenleaf, and Julian M. Davidson, "Plasma Oxytocin Increases in the Human Sexual Response, *Journal of Clinical Endocrinology & Metabolism* 64, no. 1 (January 1987): 27–31.

Chapter 6

44. "Outliers," *Masters of Sex*, Season 4, Episode 5.

45. Wendy Zerin, MD, personal correspondence, March 2019.

46. Author unknown, *The Illustrated Koka Shastra Medieval Indian Writings on Love Based on the Kama Sutra*, trans. Alex Comfort (New York: Simon & Shuster, 1997).

47. Sheikh Nefzawi, *The Perfumed Garden*, trans. Richard Francis Burton (UK: Dodo Press, 2005).

48. Robert L. Dickinson, *Human Sex Anatomy* (Baltimore:Williams & Wilkins, 1933), 35.

49. Betty Dodson, *Sex for One: The Joy of Selfloving* (New York: Three Rivers Press, 1974; 1983; 1987; 1996).

50. Amara Charles, *The Sexual Practices of Quodoushka: Teachings from the Nagual Tradition* (Rochester, Vermont: Destiny Books, 2011).

51. Amara Charles, personal correspondence, January 2020.

52. Sourced from Quodoushka teachings by DTMMS permission. Deer Tribe Metis Medicine Society, www.dtmms.org; www.quodoushka.org.

53. Emily Nagoski, *Come as You Are* (New York: Simon and Schuster, 2015).

54. Kelly D. Suschinsky, Jackie S. Huberman, Larah Maunder, Lori A. Brotto, Tom Hollenstein, and Meredith L. Chivers, "The Relationship between Sexual Functioning and Sexual Concordance in Women," *Journal of Sex & Marital Therapy* 45, no. 3 (March 2019): 230–46, https://doi.org/10.1080/0092 623X.2018.1518881.

55. Ferrante S. Gragasin et al., "The Neurovascular Mechanism of Clitoral Erection: Nitric Oxide and cGMP-Stimulated Activation of BKCa Channels," *FASEB Journal* 18, no 2. (September 2004): 1382–91.

Chapter 7

56. Eliot T. Berkman, "The Neuroscience of Goals and Behavior Change," *Consulting Psychology Journal 70, no. 1* (March 2018): *28–44.* https://doi.org/10.1037/cpb0000094.

57. Gaby Judah, Benjamin Gardner, Michael G. Kenward, Bianca DiStavola, and Robert Aunger, "Exploratory Study on the Impact of Perceived Reward on Habit Formation," *BMC Psychology* 6, no. 62 (2018), https://doi.org/10.1186/s40359-018-0270-z.

58. Martha Beck, *The Four-Day Win: End Your Diet War and Achieve Thinner Peace* (New York: Rodale Press, 2008).

59. Phillipa Lally, Cornelia H. M. van Jaarsveld, Henry W. W. Potts, and Jane Wardle, "How Are Habits Formed: Modelling Habit Formation in the Real World," *European Journal of Social Psychology* 40, no. 6 (October 2010): 998–1009.

60. Serena Corsini-Munt, Kate M. Rancourt, Justin P. Dubé, Meghan A. Rossi, and Natalie O. Rosen, "Vulvodynia: A Consideration of Clinical and Methodological Research Challenges and Recommended Solutions," *Journal of Pain Research* 10 (October 2017): 2425–36, https://doi.org/10.2147/JPR.S126259.

61. Not a direct quote, but information in this note was sourced from Beverly Whipple, "Ejaculation, Female," *Wiley Online Library*, November 17, 2014, https://doi.org/10.1002/9781118896877. wbiehs125.

62. A. A. Milne, *Winnie the Pooh* (New York: Dutton Books for Young Readers, 1926).

Chapter 8

63. Jett Psaris and Marlena S. Lyons, *Undefended Love* (Oakland, California: New Harbinger Publications, 2000).

64. *Merriam-Webster*, https://www.merriam-webster.com/dictionary/foreplay.

Chapter 9

65. Planned Parenthood, https://www.plannedparenthood.org/learn/relationships/sexual-consent.

66. Find out more at www.bettymartin.org.

67. *Merriam-Webster*, https://www.merriam-webster.com/dictionary/consent.

68. Betty Martin. Publicly available conference call recorded October 24, 2015. Available at https://bettymartin.org/wp-content/uploads/2015/03/oct-24-consent.mp3.

69. Information about Harry's work can be found at http://harry-faddis.com/.

70. Download the 3-Minute Game at https://bettymartin.org/how-to-play-the-3-minute-game/.

Chapter 10

71. Betty Martin. Personal correspondence, January 2020.

72. The Association for Psychological Science, "Harlow's Classic Studies Revealed the Importance of Maternal Contact," June 20, 2018, https://www.psychologicalscience.org/publications/observer/obsonline/harlows-classic-studies-revealed-the-importance-of-maternal-contact.html.

73. Learn more about ongoing studies at http://www.bucharestearlyinterventionproject.org/index.html.

74. Tiffany Field, "Touch for Socioemotional and Physical Well-Being: A Review," *Developmental Review* 30, no. 4 (December 2010): 367–83, https://www.sciencedirect.com/science/article/abs/pii/S0273229711000025.

75. Kathleen C. Light, Karen M. Grewen, and Janet A. Amico, "More Frequent Partner Hugs and Higher Oxytocin Levels Are Linked to Lower Blood Pressure and Heart Rate in Premenopausal Women," *Biological Psychology* 69, no. 1 (April 2005): 5–21, https://doi.org/10.1016/j.biopsycho.2004.11.002.

76. James A. Coan, Hillary S. Schaefer, and Richard J. Davidson, "Lending a Hand: Social Regulation of the Neural Response to Threat," *Psychological Science* 17, no. 12 (December 2006): 1032–9, https://doi.org/10.1111/j.1467-9280.2006.01832.x.

77. Paula Cocozza, "Are We Living through a Crisis of Touch?" *The Guardian*, March 7, 2018, https://www.theguardian.com/society/2018/mar/07/crisis-touch-hugging-mental-health-strokes-cuddles.

78. Mark Greene, "Why Men Need Platonic Touch," *Uplift*, December 1, 2019, https://upliftconnect.com/why-men-need-platonic-touch/.

79. Ralph Pawling, Peter R. Cannon, Francis P. McGlone, and Susannah C. Walker, "C-Tactile Afferent Stimulating Touch

Carries a Positive Affective Value," *PLoS ONE* 12, no. 3 (March 2017): e0173457, https://doi.org/10.1371/journal.pone.0173457.

80. Noel Langley, Judy Garland, Frank Morgan, Mervyn LeRoy, Florence Ryerson, Jack Haley, Ray Bolger, et al., *The Wizard of Oz* (Hollywood, California: Metro Goldwyn Mayer, 1939).

Dee Hartmann and Elizabeth Wood

Author Bios

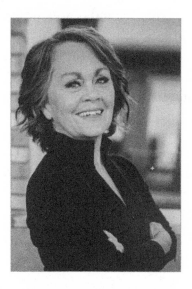

Dee Hartmann, PT, DPT

Dee earned a degree in physical therapy from Northwestern University Physical Therapy. followed by a doctor of physical therapy degree from St. Ambrose University. As part of her participation in the American Physical Therapy Association's Section on Women's Health, Dee served as the originating chairperson of the task force responsible for creating the Certificate of Achievement in Pelvic Physical Therapy. She also served on the Vulvar Pain Task Force and co-authored their findings.

A pioneer in her field, Dee is or has been a member, fellow, president, and board director for a vast array of organizations dedicated to women's sexual health and pelvic pain, including the International Pelvic Pain Society, the International Society for the

Study of Vulvovaginal Disease, and the International Society for the Study of Women's Sexual Health. Her research and findings are widely published in journals and books. She has been a guest lecturer and instructor at numerous schools, universities, workshops, and conferences around the world.

As a sole practitioner, Dee used a functional perspective to help patients decrease pelvic pain and restore health. At the Center for Genital Health and Education, she continues to research sexual pain. With an added focus on pleasure, Dee brings much-needed, progressive insight into educating people through VulvaLove, Inc., a company she founded together with Elizabeth Wood.

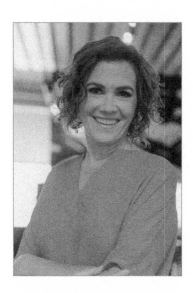

Elizabeth Wood, MSW, CSSE, BC

Elizabeth holds a master's degree in social work and was a sex therapist for many years. She is a sought-after speaker and guest lecturer who infuses pleasure into all of her talks. She is a member of the American Association of Sexuality Educators, Counselors, and Therapists and the Sexual and Gender Health Collaborative of the Front Range.

Elizabeth is a certified tantra educator, somatic sex educator, and sexological bodyworker, allowing her to work masterfully with her clients utilizing a hands-on approach. Her most recent certification, and, as she says, her last, is as an Erotic Blueprint Coach™ enabling her to help clients dive deeper into understanding the keys that unlock their unique turn-on.

Elizabeth and Dee kicked off the Pleasure Movement as a way for women to spread pleasure across the globe. In addition, they founded VulvaLove and the Center for Genital Health and Education to raise awareness, provide education, and conduct independent research on matters relating to genital pleasure and pain.